DEADLY
HEALTHCARE

James Dunbar | Prasuna Reddy | Stephen May

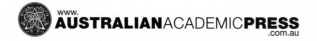

www.AUSTRALIANACADEMICPRESS.com.au

First published in 2011
Australian Academic Press
32 Jeays Street
Bowen Hills Qld 4006
Australia
www.australianacademicpress.com.au

National Library of Australia Cataloguing-in-Publication entry:

Author:	Dunbar, James A.
Title:	Deadly healthcare / James Dunbar, Prasuna Reddy, Stephen May
Edition:	1st ed.
ISBN:	9781921513756 (pbk.)
	9781921513763 (ebook)
Notes:	Includes index.
Subjects:	Patel, Jayant.
	Bundaberg Base Hospital.
	Physicians--Malpractice--Queensland--Bundaberg.
Other Authors/ Contributors:	Reddy, Prasuna, 1956-
	May, Stephen, 1961-
Dewey Number:	610.99432.

Cover photograph by © iStockphoto/VlaKol; image of Jayant Patel by © AP Images/Tertius Pickard.
Cover design by Maria Biaggini.

A thoroughly enjoyable read. With fascinating detail the authors clearly demonstrate the thin veneer covering all healthcare systems. There are lessons to be learned from this case by all countries.

This well-researched and racily written account is a cautionary tale about what can happen in the crunch of tight budgets, staff shortages and purblind hospital administrations. The risks of another Patel will increase unless the lessons from this case are well learned. It is an essential and riveting read.

A compellingly written story of serious harm. A deep understanding of quality improvement enables the authors to identify systemic failures that enhanced individual failure. They draw on international examples of similar events to demonstrate powerfully how we shouldn't allow these things to happen — but warn we are not learning the lessons. This should be compulsory reading for managers, clinicians and politicians.

Drawing on the disciplines of medicine and psychology, this insightful and compelling story examines Patel's personal narrative as well as the political and professional environment that led to the Bundaberg Hospital becoming an accident waiting to happen.

This meticulous account of the tragic consequences of poor standards at many levels in the Australian medical system is salutary, not only for that country but throughout the world. The ability of Patel to move between three continents after attracting major problems in his surgical care is breathtaking. It is, however, probably not unique. This book deserves to be read as much by medical managers and administrators as doctors.

Professor R Hugh MacDougall, Dean of the Faculty of Medicine and Head of the School of Medicine, University of St Andrews.

Critically, the events described in graphic detail in this book are not unique to Bundaberg Hospital in Queensland, but are relevant to hospitals everywhere. This book should be regularly read by every clinician, hospital executive and, above all, every health bureaucrat, to remind them of what can occur when standards of quality and safety in patient care are compromised.

Professor Alan Wolff, Director of Medical Services, Wimmera Health Care Group, Horsham, Australia.

The United Kingdom has over recent decades had its own fair share of inquiries into failing services and poorly performing healthcare professionals that have been 'covered up' by acts of both omission and commission in the healthcare organisations they have worked in. This book demonstrates why investigators and regulators need to be independent from the organisations and institutions they oversee to avoid complicity with the events they are investigating. Good governance systems can be made to work in different organisational configurations provided that there is appropriate external scrutiny or quality assurance of those systems and, importantly, local owner-ship of delivering high quality care.

Dr Frances M Elliot, Chief Executive, NHS Quality Improvement Scotland.

James Dunbar, a respected medical educator and leader in healthcare safety quality, with able support from his fellow authors, brings acute observational skills to bear on the infamous 'Dr Death' episode that shook the public's trust in the health system of the State of Queensland and changed the healthcare regulatory environment in Australia. This book is a concise and very readable account of the many underlying issues in the saga that cascaded together with disastrous consequences for patients. It starkly underlines the lessons that must be learned to keep patients safe.

Bruce Barraclough, AO, FRACS, and former President, International Society for Quality in Health Care and of the Royal Australasian College of Surgeons.

This is a gripping treatise on the collision of individual ego, organisational incompetence and political mendacity. The authors have used their considerable experience of medicine and organisations to identify a range of sobering explanations for a series of recent medical disasters. Within the text is a fascinating analysis of psychological factors which, had they been understood and acted upon, might have prevented the unfolding of one of medicine's greatest scandals. This is a story that illustrates that the road to healthcare hell is paved with good intentions — but also with potholes of bureaucratic and political incompetence. Along with the authors, I was left wondering whether sick health care institutions were capable of real recovery.

Dr Don Coid, BM, FRCPEd, and former Chief
Administrative Medical Officer, NHS Tayside, Scotland.

Table of Contents

Acknowledgments

Over the course of the five or so years of interviews, communication and research that went into this book, the authors have been provided with invaluable help. We would like to acknowledge in particular the following people for their time, stories, ideas and inspiration: Dr Bill Beresford, Beryl Crosby, Judge Geoffrey Davies AO, Dr Stephen Duckett, Dr Bill Glasson, Glennis Goodman, Toni Hoffman, Dr Harry McConnell, Rob Messenger MP, Anthony Morris QC, Dr Denis Muller, Associate Professor Kerry Petersen, Dr Martin Strahan, Dr John Wakefield, Professor Michael Ward, Professor Lyndon Wing, Don Colburn, Professor Sir Graeme Catto, Professor Sir Neil Douglas, Dr Frances Elliot, Professor Stuart Emslie, Professor R. Hugh MacDougall, Sir John Oldham, Dr Arvind Kotecha, Dr RT Mehta, and Dr Mansurali Mumdani.

About the Authors

Professor James Dunbar (MD, FRCPEdin, FRCGP, FRACGP, FFPHM) is the inaugural Director of the Greater Green Triangle University Department of Rural Health, Flinders and Deakin Universities, Australia. His main research interests are in diabetes, heart disease and depression from prevention through to better management in primary care. He also has a long-standing interest in the contribution of organisational development to improve performance in primary care. In his former post of Medical Director of Borders Primary Care NHS Trust in Scotland, he won the Golden Phoenix Award — the primary award for improvement in health care in the UK.

Professor Prasuna Reddy (PhD, MAPs) is Chair of Rural Mental Health Flinders University, and Director of Research, Greater Green Triangle University Department of Rural Health. She is a practising health and organisational psychologist, and her areas of expertise are applied psychology in health systems, and professional ethics. Professor Reddy was also coordinator of the Ethics Law and Professional Development program at Deakin University School of Medicine until mid-2009, and a member of the Human Research Ethics Committee of the Department of Human Services Victoria. She is currently Director of *Training for Life! Taking Action on Diabetes* a joint initiative of the Victorian Government and Diabetes Australia — Victoria.

Stephen May (BSc Hons) originally trained as a psychologist, but left the profession to establish his own publishing company. He published Australia's first professional magazine of psychology from 1988 to 1990, contributing numerous feature articles, interviewing psychologists and profiling psychological research and issues across the country. He has edited an extensive range of scientific and professional books as well as written for newspapers on psychological topics. He is currently President of the Australian Publishers Association.

1

Dr Death

It was a newspaper editor's dream. A cracking good story, complete with gory details, bad guys, heroes, cover-ups, whistleblowers, death, mayhem and family tragedy, and above all an evil villain — the mysterious 'Dr Death'.

For most of 2005, and again in 2010, Australian papers, radio and television ran heavily with the unfolding drama of a foreign-trained surgeon called Jayant Patel who since 2003 had appeared to be killing his patients through ineptness at a regional public hospital in Queensland.

Yet early attempts by hospital staff to reveal the unfolding disaster were seemingly being blocked by hospital management and government health bureaucrats. Patel was strongly defended and his accusers publicly ridiculed. The authorities said the whole affair was nothing more than 'a clash of personalities'.

The early news reports, however, told of staff hiding patients from a surgeon bent on carrying out complex, dangerous and sometimes unnecessary medical procedures at an under resourced and overworked hospital. Grieving parents and partners told of the traumatic deaths of their loved ones.

An investigative journalist named Hedley Thomas from Queensland's major daily newspaper, *The Courier-Mail*, blew the lid right off the story when he revealed that Patel had already been banned from performing surgery in the US after a formal review of three cases where his patients ended up dead. The Oregon Board of Medical Examiners had restricted Patel's right to practise in 2000, and the New York Medical Board had requested the surrendering of his licence to practise in that state as well in April 2001. But there was more. A trail of restrictions, censures and probations involving Patel's medical practice apparently stretched back to 1984. And Thomas had discovered all of this from a simple Google search.

Suddenly, everyone was asking how in the world such a surgeon got into a country that prides itself on its high standard of free public medical care, was registered, given a job, and left to operate unsupervised with such horrific consequences. As the accusations flew and the heroes and villains were lined up by the media for public adoration or condemnation, Patel himself was allowed to leave the country. Soon the spotlight fell on the Queensland public healthcare system which was starting to look like a very sick body in need of its own life-saving treatment.

The outcry forced the Queensland Government to set up a formal inquiry. But soon after the inquiry had begun to take evidence its head was sensationally sacked after two managers of the hospital at the centre of the controversy successfully challenged him for perceived bias. Public pressure soon forced the establishment of a second inquiry. All the while the nation's media was a battleground where the government, the whistleblowers and the victims fought for airtime and their own point of view. The inquiry finally brought down its conclusions in November 2005.

Jayant Patel was accused of being responsible for at least 48 serious adverse medical outcomes resulting in at least 13 deaths while in the employ of the Queensland Government. Yet blame was spread further than the rogue surgeon himself. Doctors, administrators, bureaucrats and politicians were all featured in a gallery of those who must take responsibility as determined by the inquiries. There were criminal charges, sackings and demotions. There was even a third inquiry — this time into the Queensland Government healthcare system itself.

Meanwhile Jayant Patel was being pursued by Australian journalists who travelled to his home town of Portland, Oregon, in the US. Filing stories kerbside outside of his home, they kept the Australian public primed for sensational news and the Queensland Government under pressure to extradite him back to Australia for trial. One news crew even managed to catch Patel in a Portland store carpark while getting back into his SUV after buying a lottery ticket. He refused to answer any questions.

In July 2008 Australian authorities succeeded in their extradition efforts and Patel arrived in Brisbane to face trial on 14 offences including three counts of manslaughter, one of causing grievous bodily harm and one of committing negligent acts causing harm. He was convicted on 29 June 2010 of three counts of manslaughter and one count of grievous bodily harm and sentenced to imprisonment, the first such conviction in Australia of medical manslaughter since 1843.

Patel's legal team immediately lodged an appeal, claiming that judicial rulings during the trial had resulted in a miscarriage of justice. But only a couple of months later Patel ran out of money to pay his counsel, and, refused the option of legal aid, was only able to get his appeal reinstated with the support of a high profile barrister working pro bono. The Queensland Government, still obviously smarting over the whole affair, immediately lodged their own appeal arguing that the seven-year sentence was in fact too lenient. Claim and counter claim was heard by three senior judges of the Queensland Court of Appeal who eventually concluded on April 21 2011 in a unanimous rejection of both appeals that Patel had suffered no miscarriage of justice and that his sentence was appropriate.

The tale of Jayant Patel and his time at Bundaberg Hospital under the employ of the Queensland Government is much more than a tragic story from a busy rural hospital. It is a dramatic warning of how things can go horribly wrong in any modern health-care system. Failure to learn from the mistakes revealed by the Patel case will ensure something like it could happen again.

Jayant Patel is no homicidal maniac intent on murder who cut a violent swath across two continents one step ahead of authorities before being caught. Nor is he a bumbling, under talented surgeon who can't hold down a job and was finally exposed and humiliated at a regional Australian hospital. Everywhere Patel has worked there are public records of both praise for and criticism of his surgical skills and professional manner. He has treated thousands of patients, most of whom suffered no ill-effects from coming into contact with him.

He appears to be a mediocre surgeon with a strong, self-absorbed, dysfunctional personality and a compulsive manner who worked in a healthcare system already strained by staff shortages, inadequate funding, poor work practices and flawed central management, until his aberrant behaviour became so deadly that it had to be stopped.

The process it took to finally convince Queensland Health to end Patel's working contract set off an avalanche of documented public analysis and information about Patel and his interaction with the various healthcare systems under which he had worked since 1978. While finally exposed as the danger he is from his time in Australia, the fact remains that Patel had been duly registered and permitted to treat patients across three health jurisdictions in the US — New York, Pennsylvania and Oregon — before unleashing his deadly version of healthcare on the Australian public. He had already been sanctioned, struck off, and his medical conduct critically examined by professionals.

Ploughing through the mass of public inquiry data and interviewing key figures in the affair reveals that the story of Jayant Patel and his time at Bundaberg is symptomatic of a tidal wave that is heading towards all modern healthcare systems. Each system in comparable countries will soon be competing with every other system because of international workforce shortages. As the population ages, there will be a smaller working population and a reducing pool of people choosing to work in healthcare. Meanwhile, advances in medical technology and treatment will ensure hospitals remain expensive organisations to run. The pressure to ensure that the medical workforce is well trained and safe and continues to perform its medical duties with the utmost emphasis on patient care will be increasingly compromised by the pressures of staff shortages and the need to manage financial considerations. This is a recipe that can bring about institutional weaknesses able to be exploited by individuals with serious personality problems just like Jayant Patel.

There is no way of predicting when and where another Patel will surface, but it is clear that the trust the public places in modern healthcare is based on the assumption that the system includes adequate patient safety. Mistakes will happen, but it is assumed that individuals within an organisation are supported by an administrative structure that will allow malpractice to be revealed quickly and investigated efficiently and impartially.

The story of what happened at Bundaberg Hospital is not just a scary bedtime read to be put down at its conclusion with the reader secure in the knowledge that the villain has been captured and put to justice. It is a wake-up call to governments and the community to learn from the tragic events how to be better at protecting patients.

2

'Dazed and distressed'

You could already feel the heat of the day to come by 7 am on September 2005 as we arrived at Queensland's Bundaberg Base Hospital to interview Dr Bill Beresford, the newly installed head of the hospital now known throughout Australia and beyond as the workplace of 'Dr Death' aka Dr Jayant Patel. Here we would begin to examine a complex set of failures, oversights and poor health management practices that allowed the entry of a rogue surgeon into the hospital with catastrophic results.

Beresford had recently retired as Director of Medical Services of the Royal Perth Hospital on Australia's west coast and had been spending time with his grandchildren in the UK fending off job offers. A highly respected hospital administrator, Beresford was in constant demand. But it was the urgent and persistent approach from the Deputy Director General of Queensland Health that persuaded him to cut short his holiday and return to Australia.

The Queensland Government needed the hospital fixed. The carnage left by Patel also brought with it significant collateral damage to the main players in the tragedy. Patel faced numerous criminal charges including fraud, grievous bodily harm, and manslaughter. The Bundaberg Hospital Executive Director of Medical Services also faced criminal charges. The Bundaberg District Manager had been referred to a state Crime and Misconduct Commission, and there were resignations and sackings, including a government Health Minister, one Departmental Director General and two Deputy Directors General.

Beresford's new job was to rebuild a shattered hospital, re-establishing the lost faith of a local population shocked by several months of public inquiries revealing frightening tales of medical incompetence and cover-up. His task was to make the hospital a safe place once again.

Beresford hails from Patley Bridge, a small village in North Yorkshire, England, and still has the blunt, accented speech of his native county. Of medium height and build, with a full head of greying hair, he speaks slowly and deliberately, often with his eyes closed when concentrating. Not given to speculation, he takes a forensic approach to the facts and will not accept or give a statement without evidence.

He is a good listener, a reflective but straightforward man who demonstrates his moral authority to his audience. They know that what he says will come to pass.

He is also no stranger to the debilitating effects on staff morale and personal functioning that a major health inquiry into a hospital can produce, having served previously as a medical director following an official health inquiry into hospital activities at King Edward Memorial Hospital in Perth. It was one of the reasons he was chosen for the job. He already knew what to expect as he entered Bundaberg Hospital. He described it to us as akin to Stalingrad in 1944. Almost all the infrastructure was in ruins and the people emerged from these ruins dazed and distressed. With top managers stood aside or on sick leave, the organisational memory, policies and procedures were lost. Paradoxically, when you most want to make a hospital safe, it is the hardest time to do it.

Beresford knew that he had to rebuild the hospital by first getting the confidence and trust of everyone there. His approach was to tour the clinical areas of the hospital daily, talking to everyone before arriving in his office at 9 am. This is a man who leads by 'walking the job' like an old style Medical Superintendent. He relies on human contact.

Hospital staff quickly learnt what time he should be passing by each morning. Slowly they started to tell him more and more about what was happening in the hospital. Beresford described it as 'like dealing with a wounded dog'. After what people had been through, staff looked for someone who listens to them, understands their problems, develops plans for the future and shares a vision of a much-improved Bundaberg Hospital.

The wider community is divided in the aftermath of Patel. Many locals work for the hospital, each with family and relations deeply concerned about and interested in what happens there. There are those who, like nurse Toni Hoffman, a major whistleblower in the entire affair, saw Patel as a dangerously incompetent surgeon. Others sided with management's defence of him. Following the allegations about his poor surgical record, the patients have become divided too. There are those who definitely had adverse consequences from his surgery, those who might wonder if they had too, and others who simply feel involved despite a tenuous and distance relationship with Patel. The number of patients who feel themselves affected by Patel's work is well out of proportion to reality and has generated an additional set of problems.

'It is like unresolved grief', said Beresford. 'All sorts of bad things need to go into the casket before it can be removed from the hospital and buried.' It was a process that would take a long time. In the meantime, many of the staff leaders from both factions of opinion were on stress leave, adding a further burden to the hospital.

Yet the effects were wider than just at the hospital. Dr Martin Strahan, former Director of Medicine at Bundaberg, saw the fallout from the immense surge of publicity surrounding the case that swamped Australia's news and current affairs outlets for months. He felt it had brought about a general decline in confidence in the medical profession in the Bundaberg area, and wider: 'Patel betrayed a trust, and the consequences of that have been bad for the patients and they have been bad for Bundaberg, but in a sense it has sort of rocked the whole of the medical profession in Australia.'

Bundaberg Base Hospital wasn't always an accident waiting to happen. It has a long history of providing essential healthcare to the predominantly rural population of the Wide Bay district that surrounds the Burnett River. Set in the middle of a town on a flat alluvial plain providing excellent soil conditions for farming, 'the Base' as it is sometimes referred to by locals is the only public hospital in Bundaberg alongside the two private facilities of the Friendly Society Private Hospital and the Mater Hospital.

Bisected by the river, Bundaberg is a mixture of a few architecturally significant historical buildings and an expanse of low, drab and monotonous structures dominated by the smoking stacks of the local rum distillery which produces the popular 'Bundaberg Rum' brand. The population is largely Anglo-Celtic, with a few Chinese and a tiny Indian community almost entirely employed at the hospital.

The hospital began its life in 1880 as a four-room cottage with a separate kitchen and single ward to treat the medical ailments of the blackbirded Melanesian workers known as Kanakas who toiled on the area's vast cane fields. In 1914 this had expanded into a formal state hospital with new buildings opened by the then Queensland Governor, Sir William McGregor, forming the core of the present day complex on Bourbong Street. By 1994, the district's population had grown to 80,000 and Bundaberg Hospital was a busy place. It had 140 beds and a staff of 850 including 65 doctors and an annual budget of $62 million, serving a population of about 85,000 and receiving 18,000 admissions, 24,500 outpatients and 28,500 emergency patients each year.

The state government department responsible for public hospitals, Queensland Health, headquartered 385 kilometres south in Brisbane, managed Bundaberg and 177 other public hospitals across Australia's most decentralised state, where 48 per cent of the population live outside major cities. The department had an illustrious history, being the first in Australia to provide a free and universal public hospital system in the 1940s. But recently it had fallen on tougher times, coming to rely on overseas trained doctors to fill a growing shortfall. Many rural hospitals had begun to feel under resourced. But they carried on as best they could.

The newly appointed Director of Medical Services at Bundaberg Hospital was a vascular surgeon called Brian Thiele. He grew up in Bundaberg, married a local girl, trained in Victoria, Australia, and worked as a surgeon in the US for 18 years. In 1994, as he approached retirement, he decided to leave his position as Head Surgeon at Pennsylvania State University Hospital and return to Bundaberg.

He was known as a 'hands-on' leader who toured a portion of the hospital every Friday with the Director of Nursing, Glennis Goodman, and also ran his own clinic. Thiele believed that the only way to be sure a hospital was running well was by walking around to see for yourself. As a strong supporter of the value of education for the maintenance of clinical standards, he introduced weekly clinical meetings, visits from Brisbane specialists, and regular educational presentations. He got on well with the hospital's District Manager, Bruce Marshall, the Director of Medicine, Dr Martin Strahan, and the Director of Surgery, Dr Pitre Anderson, and felt that it was important to create an environment that attracted good medical resident officers. His efforts were rewarded in the mid-1990s when the Australian and New Zealand College of Surgeons granted training accreditation to the hospital that allowed it to attract medical registrars from Brisbane hospitals. Thiele always felt that registrars were important to the hospital because of their high level of competence, their ability to take the load off specialists, and the fact that they would eventually be able to progress to become specialists themselves in other regional hospitals. He also encouraged strong links with the local community, liaising with Bundaberg business leaders about providing funding for the hospital.

Overall, professional life at the hospital once Thiele began his tenure benefited immensely. There was a clear sense of camaraderie and positivity among the staff despite ongoing frustration with increasingly centralised decisions from Queensland Health. There were regular staff barbeques, dinners and even a Christmas pageant. Social interaction out of hours between visiting medical officers and the full-time specialist staff was common. The District Manager would even sometimes join the festivities, allowing the opportunity to be quizzed by senior doctors on wider professional and medical management issues. The hospital was able to establish an important new renal service and remained focused on what was in the interest of the local community. Surgeons would run long operating lists and look after large numbers of patients efficiently and happily. Productivity was high. The staff felt that, though under resourced and subject to whatever missives came out of Queensland Health, Bundaberg Hospital belonged to the people of the area and would not be stopped from doing something that they felt should be done for the local health needs of the Wide Bay and Burnett regions.

For Theile, the next five years spent as Director of Medical Services at Bundaberg Hospital saw everything unwind, as his work-place became a battlefield — leading to a complete capitulation in the face of a progressive loss of registrar doctors and a decline in patient care that was out of his control. What started as a joyous return home to a professional role practising caring and compas-sionate medicine to his local community turned into a nightmarish conflict with Queensland Health.

Thiele saw Queensland Health as obsessive in exerting control from head office at the expense of local control and autonomy. The department seemed opposed to engaging visiting medical officers whom they could not control and preferred instead salaried staff. The department seemed to him to be heavily politicised and full of

professional administrators rather than clinicians, who were reluctant to discuss issues relating to levels of patient care such as long
waiting lists and the absence of vital medical equipment. When the
department did respond to Thiele's concerns, they downplayed their
importance in the light of budgetary concerns.

In Thiele's view, the local district health councils that were sup-
posed to look out for such problems were powerless and only given
filtered information. Queensland Health also failed to implement a
detailed study of the need for clinical services at the hospital and
instead budgets continued to be based on a purely historical basis.
There was no attempt to match the budgets to clinical standards or
demographic trends. Each year Queensland Health would fix the
budget centrally and expect Bundaberg Hospital to work within it.

To Thiele, the department seemed intent on reducing responsibility for personal patient care and replacing it with an imposed uniformity and a form-based assessment approach that could be linked
directly back to cost efficiency. When a Queensland Health directive
came through from Brisbane that patients were now to be referred
to as 'clients' in line with the new corporate culture adopted for the
department, Thiele nearly exploded.

As time wore on, these issues were discussed vigorously at the
monthly meetings of the Medical Staff Advisory Committee.
Through the completion of quality assurance questionnaires that
went to Queensland Health, they made comments such as 'care is
delivered on an *ad hoc* basis as continuum of care is impossible
within current staffing levels … management appear more interested in making targets than delivery of quality healthcare', and
'management continues to ignore safe working hours, practices and
the fact that the anaesthetics department is grossly understaffed.'
Despite the scathing nature of these comments, neither the hospital
management nor Queensland Health sought clarification.

Dr Thiele resigned in March 1999, moving to a two-day-a-week
Visiting Medical Officer position before leaving the hospital entirely
in 2003.

Queensland Health continued to push hard and everyone was feeling the pinch.

Dr Chris Jelliffe worked for two years at Bundaberg as an anaesthetist while converting his British Fellowship of the Royal College of Anaesthetists to its Australian equivalent. While another anaesthetist was on study leave in 2002, Jelliffe was forced to be on call for eight days straight as the only full-time anaesthetist responsible for emergencies, obstetrics, intensive care and elective surgery. He became severely fatigued, suffered sleep disturbances and believed his judgment was becoming impaired. He felt that his condition could compromise patient safety and cancelled any elective surgery that could be delayed. He immediately notified the Director of Medical Services of the decision and was called to the District Manager's office the same day. Instead of finding his attitude to patient care being supported, the District Manager none too subtly reminded him of his work visa status which was tied to his Queensland Health contract as an Overseas Trained Doctor. Jelliffe construed this as a threat and soon looked for work elsewhere.

Glennis Goodman has worked at Bundaberg Hospital for 25 years. Around this time she recalls the hospital being a million dollars over budget and visited by a Queensland Health manager from Brisbane who pressured the then District Manager, Peter Leck, so much that Leck went into the next hospital executive meeting and declared: 'You will lose your jobs if you do not bring this budget in.'

The hospital also lost two successive directors of surgery. Pitre Anderson, Thiele's replacement, stepped down in 2000 when standards began to slip below those set by the Royal Australasian College of Surgeons. Those standards include caseload education programs, supervision of junior medical staff, and audit and peer review processes. Anderson eventually found himself with an excessive workload and lack of support from management. Even when Anderson took the extreme step of going public about the dangers of overworked surgeons he found himself personally attacked under parliamentary privilege by the then Queensland Health Minister,

Wendy Edmond. He remained at Bundaberg as another Visiting Medical Officer, and Anderson's replacement, colleague Dr Charles Nankivell who had started at Bundaberg in 1995, soon found he had been passed a poisoned chalice.

Nankivell and Anderson had been working a dangerous one-in-two roster due to staff shortages. With such a roster, if one doctor is on leave, the other might be on call for 19 days straight. By this time the hospital had no other surgeons on staff so, when Anderson resigned, Nankivell had the 'shattering experience' of being the only surgeon available for almost three months. Queensland Health did nothing to relieve the situation or remunerate him for the extra time he worked.

Nankivell kept trying to convince Queensland Health of the declining standard of patient care at the hospital, but was increasingly feeling it was a worthless effort. He was talking to bureaucrats, not clinicians. The department quality assurance systems were all about finances not medical standards. Going over budget was considered by the bureaucratic managers as an instant failure of a KPI (key performance indicator), instead of a possible indication that the budget might need to be revised in the light of medical requirements.

Queensland Health seemingly did not welcome complaints about such matters. Instead, Nankivell felt that people tended to get sacked for disagreeing. Nevertheless, he persisted in providing evidence of the deteriorating standard of care and even suggested it could still be resolved in part by employing visiting medical officers from two small private hospitals in the region. Queensland Health disagreed with this approach and maintained that financially things were better by just employing two full-time surgeons. By the end of 2001, Nankivell had had enough. As well as the stress of his job he had a wife and two young children. He was spending nearly every day at the hospital. He left in January the next year. No attempt was made by Queensland Health to talk him out of his resignation.

Between November 2001 and August 2002, Dr Sam Baker filled the post of Director of Surgery. Like Nankivell, he had grave concerns that the hospital management were putting budget concerns ahead of patient safety. There was now inadequate supervision of junior doctors in the emergency department and Queensland Health was slow to replace staff even when it resulted in surgeons being on call continuously for days. Baker couldn't help thinking this was a deliberate cost cutting exercise. He was already well used to hospital roster changes and operating procedures directed from Brisbane that came with a supporting 'business case' and concomitant detailed financial savings. He, too, was not timid in voicing his concerns and spoke out publicly about Nankivell's resignation. He immediately received a 'please explain' from District Manager Peter Leck. Baker resigned and left Bundaberg in September 2002.

With the departure of Baker, Dr Lakshman Jayasekera moved up as acting Director of Surgery. Jayasekera had been employed as the hospital's required second full-time surgeon following Nankivell's departure. He was a Sri Lankan graduate with a Fellowship of the Royal College of Surgeons of Edinburgh. When he migrated to Australia in 1996 he obtained Fellowship of the Royal Australasian College of Surgeons.

By this time the hospital had also employed Dr Anatoli Kotlovsky, a Russian paediatric surgeon whose qualifications were not recognised in Australia. He had worked as a non-accredited surgical registrar and never been employed as a surgeon in Australia and therefore was required under the terms of his registration to be supervised. This now brought Bundaberg Hospital to the point where it no longer had the two Fellows of the Royal Australasian College of Surgeons required to continue its registrar training status. Without the registrars, and with already overworked surgical staff, a further substantial reduction in quality of care was the only outcome that could be expected.

Dr Kees Nydam, acting Director of Medical Services at the time, advertised in August for yet another Director of Surgery. The advertisement said that the applicant should have 'qualifications as a general surgeon acceptable for specialist registration by the Medical

Board'. Nydam encouraged Dr Jayasekera to apply. There were two other applicants for the post and Dr Jayasekera was short-listed along with Dr Boris Strekozov to be interviewed by a selection panel consisting of Nydam, Leck the District Manager, and Anderson. The post was offered to Dr Strekozov but after some weeks of consideration he rejected the offer. Surprisingly the position was not offered to Jayasekera, though Queensland Health guidelines would have allowed such an event. Instead the position was advertised again. But this time there were no applications. Jayasekera continued to indicate that he would accept the position if it was offered even though he was still seeking to move closer to his family in Brisbane. No offer was forthcoming. Jayasekera felt humiliated and gave three months notice of intention to resign from 28 December 2002.

It is clear that overlooking Jayasekera was a source of tension between senior doctors and management. The minutes of a Medical Staff Advisory Committee endorsed by six doctors stated that the meeting accepted the resignation of Dr Jayasekera with great regret and that 'this is one of many resignations leading to the effective demise of General Surgery at the Bundaberg Hospital ... largely due to the dictatorial, unresponsive, myopic and inflexible approach of management who have little regard for specialists, their needs, or aspirations'. Both Nydam and Leck were asked to explain to the meeting why Dr Jayasekera had not been offered the position, but did not respond. Jayasekera left the hospital in March 2003.

The hospital was at this stage still short two surgeons, with one required to fulfil the position of Director of Surgery, but Nydam now only advertised for a Senior Medical Officer, Surgery. The sole qualifications required were that the applicant had experience in surgical services, and could be registered as a medical practitioner. It did not require specialist qualifications in general surgery. The position description did, however, state that the successful applicant would report directly to the Director of Surgery. Yet there was in fact no Director of Surgery at the hospital.

One of the recipients of Nydam's advertisement was Wavelength International, a Sydney-based company that recruits doctors from overseas in return for a commission equivalent to 15 per cent of the doctor's first-year salary package. Wavelength had a number of US doctors on their books interested in working in Australia, including Dr Jayant Patel, then unemployed for some 15 months after leaving the employ of Kaiser Permanente in Portland, Oregon.

Patel's CV was passed on to Nydam. It stated that he was a US citizen, Fellow of the American College of Surgeons, and a general surgeon with some experience in paediatric, vascular and general surgery. It included six open references at least a year old, four of which came from former work colleagues in Portland. There was no explanation as to why Patel had left his previous employment and why he wanted to work in Australia. Wavelength had contacted two of the referees, who both confirmed good references for Patel.

Nydam also surprisingly received a second US applicant from Wavelength, Dr James Gaffield, who had a special interest in plastic surgery. Delighted that he now had the prospect of filling both vacant surgery positions right away, Nydam recommended the two surgeons be offered jobs but felt Patel was the superior candidate to Gaffield and would be better suited as Director of Surgery, although that was a position Patel could not be appointed to without being a member of the Royal Australasian College of Surgeons.

By all accounts, Nydam was thrilled to finally be receiving not one, but two US surgeons. Senior hospital staff began to feel that their long efforts in sending submissions for more staff down to Brisbane had been taken notice of.

Wavelength then set about arranging for the doctors to obtain registration with the Queensland Medical Board and securing visas from the Department of Immigration and Ethnic Affairs. Patel's application for registration in Queensland included the following questions: Have you been registered under the *Medical Practitioners' Registration Act 2001* or the *Medical Act 1939* (repealed) or have you been registered under a corresponding law applying, or that applied in another state, or territory, or a foreign country, and that registration was effective either by an undertaking, the imposition of a condition, suspension or cancellation in any other way? Has your registration as a health practitioner ever been cancelled or suspended or is your registration currently cancelled or suspended as a result of disciplinary action in any state or territory or in any other country?

To each of these questions, Patel answered 'No'. He faxed off the Oregon Medical Board's verification of licensure to Wavelength and mailed the original. The documents included a sentence that read: 'Standing: public order on file — see attached.' Patel did not include the attachment in either the faxed or mailed material.

The Queensland Medical Board duly assessed the documents passed on by Wavelength and at a meeting of the Registration Advisory Committee meeting on 3 February 2003 agreed that Patel ought not to be represented as a specialist but recommended that he be approved under a special purpose registration to fill an Area of Need as a registered Staff Medical Officer (SMO) under the supervision of the Director of Surgery. Gaffield would be employed as a general surgeon. Both these positions still required that the doctors would report to the still non-existent Director of Surgery. Patel would arrive first, Gaffield about a month later.

Yet, by the time Patel arrived, his position at Bundaberg had been elevated by Nydam to that of the vacant Director of Surgery, a position for which Patel had not applied, and which was clearly inconsistent with the terms of the registration that had been granted to him by the Medical Board.

On 1 April 2003, Glennis Goodman took the opportunity to greet Patel on his first day at Bundaberg Hospital. The Director of Nursing Services warmly introduced herself and told Patel she hoped he would enjoy his stay in Bundaberg. His reply struck her as peculiar and demeaning: 'Yes, well, we've all got to do our stint in a third world country.'

Dr Patel had arrived.

3

'Doctors don't have germs'

Jayant Patel wasted little time getting into the operating theatre. He was now the only full-time surgeon at the hospital, with no surgical supervisor or even another staff surgeon with whom to consult and confer. To Patel, that didn't seem a problem.

On 19 May 2003 Patel performed his first oesophagectomy at Bundaberg on a 46-year-old male patient, James Phillips, who was already suffering kidney failure and requiring dialysis. The operation was to remove a lesion by cutting away a portion of his oesophagus. The need for dialysis complicated the procedure greatly and there was some prior discussion about transferring the patient to a specialist unit at a large Brisbane hospital. Patel went ahead anyway. Phillips survived the operating theatre but was wheeled into the intensive care unit in an unstable and dangerous state. Despite the best efforts of the ICU staff, he died sometime later.

Nurse Unit Manager of the Intensive Care Unit, Toni Hoffman, was deeply worried about this incident. Not that patients don't die in hospitals — ICUs are places where severely sick people are cared for — some don't make it. She was concerned that the operation was not appropriate for their limited resources but guessed that, if it was an emergency, then it had to be done. What concerned Hoffman was whether the operation really had to be performed then and there. Patel's behaviour struck her as odd and troubling, both during the operation and afterward as the ICU staff struggled with the limited resources available to them to try and save James Phillips.

Though not a staff member with any history of making complaints to managers, Hoffman expressed her concerns to Glennis Goodman, Director of Nursing, who arranged a meeting with the new Queensland Health Director of Medical Services, Dr Darren Keating, Hoffman, and Dr John Joiner, a GP with an interest in anaesthetics.

Keating had himself only arrived in Bundaberg two weeks after Dr Patel. A 1986 graduate of the University of Melbourne, he had extensive experience in the Australian Army up to 2000 when he left to become Senior Medical Officer in Port Hedland Regional Hospital in Western Australia. He was given little training or induction at Bundaberg, describing his experience as being 'literally thrown into work straight away and learning as I went'.

Three areas of concern featured at that meeting. Hoffman said that Patel was habitually 'rude, loud, and did not work collaboratively' with ICU staff; that there was 'a whole bravado about things and things didn't match up'; and that his choice of drugs and treatment seemed to be 'twenty years behind contemporary thinking'. Hoffman also pointed out that, although the patient was extremely unwell, Patel kept telling the family and writing in clinical notes that the patient was 'stable'. She also raised the question of whether oesophagectomies should be carried out at all in the hospital because of its limited capacity for intensive care.

Despite those concerns being raised, Patel carried out a second oesophagectomy in early June. This time it was on a cancer patient and resulted in severe medical complications. Hoffman compiled a written report and e-mailed it to Keating, drawing attention to the complications, the lack of sufficient ICU back-up care, concern by

Brisbane hospitals that these procedures were being undertaken in Bundaberg, and Patel's continuing problematic behaviour which now seemed to include an unwillingness to transfer the patient to Brisbane. Joiner's view, also expressed to Keating, was that the Bundaberg ICU could not give intensive long-term support needed for oesophagectomies; that based on published evidence the hospital could not maintain its competency unless more than 30 oesophagectomies were performed per year; and that this patient indeed needed transfer to Brisbane immediately. The patient was finally transferred to the Mater Hospital in Brisbane on 20 June.

Doctors in Brisbane also had something to say about Patel's work. A senior intensive care doctor from the Mater Hospital wrote to Keating stating that he thought Bundaberg Hospital should not be undertaking oesophagectomies and especially in this case when surgery was not the best option because of the extensive spread of the cancer. He also queried the accreditation of Patel. Yet Patel would perform two more oesophagectomies before the issue was revisited.

The next complainant was the hospital's infection control coordinator, a nurse called Gail Aylmer. She noticed that Patel did not wash his hands between examining patients, even if he was handling their dressings and touching their wounds. This level of uncleanliness in a hospital setting can quickly lead to cross-infection and wound dehiscence which occurs when a surgical wound does not heal, usually due to infection or poor wound closure techniques. Aylmer spoke to Patel about the importance of infection control techniques but his behaviour did not change. Several nurses in the Department of Surgery commented that the incidence of wound dehiscence had been unusually high in the two months since he arrived. They also reported Patel as saying 'doctors don't have germs', when it was pointed out to him that he should wash his hands before beginning procedures. Aylmer investigated and found 13 reported incidents compared with the two or three that might be expected. In her report to Keating, she showed that most of the cases were Patel's.

Aylmer also noted Patel's curious behaviour in leaving the hospital buildings in his bloodied theatre attire so that he might grab a quick smoke out in the car park. She had received reliable reports that Dr Patel was in fact disparaging about the protocol designed to ensure that theatre staff did not leave the theatre complex in their surgical gear.

Patel's basic surgical technique was also commented on by nurses from the hospital's Renal Unit. An audit of all the patients who had received catheters for dialysis in 2003 found that every single patient who had a catheter placed by Patel had a complication — three had migrated, two had become infected and there was impaired outflow in one. Each of the catheters was considered to have been placed incorrectly. Three patients had required further surgical intervention, two had died and one had required an intravenous drip. A report was given to Peter Miach, Director of Medicine and renal physician at the hospital since August 2000. Miach forwarded the report to Keating. Miach also took matters into his own hands as far as he could. He chose to direct all future patients of his to be operated on to the Friendly Society Private Hospital across town. He directed that none of his patients be looked at by Patel and also let other staff know that, if any patients required surgery, to 'stay clear' of Patel.

Meanwhile a senior vascular surgeon from Brisbane, Jason Jenkins, became aware that Patel was working beyond his level of competence in vascular surgery. A number of patients had been transferred to Brisbane and he was particularly worried about the renal access patients. Jenkins approached Miach to voice his concerns and was astonished to learn that it was difficult to stop Patel because he tended to find patients in wards and operate on them without consulting Miach. This kind of behaviour is considered to be in direct contradiction to the accepted medical ethic of first gaining the permission of the attending doctor before operating. Jenkins went so far as to write a formal letter to Miach and Patel about one particularly serious complication in a patient with diabetes and renal problems.

The letter was passed on to Keating who did not appear to take the matter any further.

The previous Director of Medicine at Bundaberg, Martin Strahan, also found Patel's surgical skills wanting. He recalls examining a CAT scan result with Patel and noting that Patel didn't seem to know what he was actually looking at. To Strahan's amazement, Patel thought the scan showed leaking medical dye from a perforated bowel when in fact he was looking at a scan of a kidney with dye resting clearly in the urinary tract. That immediately raised doubts in Strahan's mind as to the appropriateness of any approach Patel might take to manage the patient's condition. True to the form Patel was now displaying, Patel talked confidently with Strahan about a complicated and major surgical approach called Whipple's procedure. Strahan wasn't convinced. He later reminded Keating that in fact Patel was receiving very little feedback on his clinical judgements and, since he was Director of Surgery, he wasn't actually clinically responsible to anyone. He told both Keating and Miach that Patel didn't have anyone to discuss with or consult with and there was no one checking on him.

The gravity and extent of complaints about Patel were now growing rapidly, yet hospital management apparently persistently downplayed the scale of the incidents, preferring to classify them as personality conflicts. The medical staff began to grow unwilling to communicate further problems to management because of a lack of any response. Instead they all, to one extent or another, 'worked around' the problem of Patel.

That approach broadly succeeded so long as you weren't actually admitted as Patel's patient. But the odds were against you. Patel was a prodigious worker. In his time at Bundaberg he saw over 1450 patients, operated on about 1000 and conducted over 400 endoscopies. He would organise blitzes on particular procedures; for instance, performing 15 gall-bladder operations in one week. He prided himself on the speed and volume of his surgery.

Yet it wasn't the case that Patel didn't have opportunities to avoid work. He had chosen a very nice place to live at the coastal resort hamlet of Bargara, just 15 kilometres away. His apartment was situated in an ocean front five-level luxury complex with tennis courts and swimming pool. Across the road is a golf course. Sunrises over the beach at Bargara see many locals taking an early morning barefoot stroll as the early sunrays spray a glittering sparkle of light onto a calm deep blue sea. As night falls, the beach is again alive with people before finally thinning out as locals and holidaymakers alike wander off to one of the numerous restaurants and bars that dot the foreshore. According to the manager of the resort, all of this beauty was lost on Patel, who hardly ever took leisure time except on a rare visit from his family who remained for the most part back in the US. Day and night, Patel always seemed to be at the hospital.

Such a heavy workload did bring benefits, though. It seems that Patel was keenly aware of how Bundaberg Hospital was funded and the importance of maximising that funding using Queensland Health's set targets for elective surgery. When a hospital treated a patient, the funding by Queensland Health was determined by a system of 'waited separations'; that is, by reference to a predetermined code, the complexity and expense involved in any given procedure is calculated and the hospital given funding accordingly. Patel seemed to always know the waited separation of any particular procedure and he constantly told staff how valuable he was in terms of reaching surgery targets.

He was not wrong on this point. Leck, ever the responsible business manager, would later caution against moving too quickly on any complaints about Patel lest the hospital lose the financial benefits he brought it.

Through all this Patel remained an engaging if somewhat enigmatic figure about the hospital. He was variously described by patients as 'charming', 'very confident', and that he had a 'powerful personality'. Patel could be an engaging force. Nurses talked about his ability to exude confidence and charm. One of his greatest attributes was his interest in the professional development of junior doctors. He made himself available to junior staff during the day, at night, weekends and out of hours.

In February 2004, Toni Hoffman became Acting Director of Nursing while a replacement was found for Goodman. Hoffman used the opportunity to meet again with Leck and set out in some detail her concerns about the Intensive Care Unit as a result of Patel's surgery. She provided Leck with a document entitled 'ICU Issues with Ventilated Patients' summarising her concerns. There was no action taken — the complex operations and complications continued. Patel still refused to transfer patients to Brisbane, and Hoffman now heard that he had instructed junior doctors to avoid writing certain words such as 'wound dehiscence' into the medical records of his patients.

A new Director of Nursing, Linda Mulligan, was duly appointed and Hoffman immediately approached her about the problems she saw with Patel. To Hoffman, though, Mulligan's response was not helpful. She seemed to take the view that the problems were due to a personality conflict. Hoffman, increasingly frustrated and concerned at the growing toll of deaths and disasters under Patel's care, consulted the Queensland Nurses Union about what she should do. A union representative raised the concerns with Mulligan on Hoffman's behalf to no avail. Hoffman also provided Mulligan with statements from six nurses concerning one particular case.

In October 2004, Hoffman again met with Mulligan. This time she forcefully presented her concerns and followed up in writing. She was asked to come to Leck's office where she repeated her concerns and said that the union's advice was to make a complaint to the state government's Crime and Misconduct Commission or write to the Director General of the department but that she was eager to find an internal resolution provided there was an independent audit of Patel's surgery. She again followed up the meeting with a written report. Again she heard nothing.

By now, Miach's compensations for the perceived lack of surgical skill by Patel and his warnings to doctors were becoming all too noticeable. A heated exchange reportedly took place between Miach and Keating when Keating refused to acknowledge that Miach had sent him the earlier report on catheter insertions for renal dialysis. Miach sent him another copy the following day. Keating then had meetings with a number of the medical staff in which they made their criticisms of Patel's surgery known. Yet Miach himself was not interviewed, nor Patel or any of the other doctors. Keating did not call for the files or arrange for an independent surgeon to assess the information. He instead reported to Leck that Miach's catheter report was supported by 'poor data'.

But the pressure had finally grown too strong for Leck not to do anything. On 16 December Leck made a call to Queensland Health in which he proposed dealing with the complaints about Patel by enacting a general clinical review of procedures in the ICU. The officer at Queensland Health advised Leck that the review should be done by a departmental clinician, usually the Chief Health Officer, Dr Gerry FitzGerald. Leck contacted FitzGerald, providing him with a memorandum about Hoffman's concerns and arranged for FitzGerald to visit the hospital within a month to conduct a general clinical audit rather than a full investigation.

Meanwhile Keating wrote to Patel and offered him a four-year extension of his contract. Patel declined the generous offer but received a negotiated locum rate of $1150 per day for three months as an alternative. Keating still didn't want to lose him, but he was beginning to realise that the complaints couldn't be ignored anymore and prepared a set of briefing papers for Leck. The papers spoke in glowing terms of Patel's enthusiasm, commitment to teaching and several 'innovations' in operating theatre procedures. He also acknowledged Patel's 'poor patient selection', his refusal to transfer patients, poor judgement, outdated medical knowledge and a number of allegations against him regarding infection control procedures and the issue of the catheters.

Patel was finally called in to talk with Leck about the complaints against him just prior to FitzGerald's audit. Leck managed to secure an undertaking from Patel that there would no more oesophagectomies.

When FitzGerald arrived at the hospital for the ICU audit on 14 February 2005, he was not given a full list of complaints about Patel. His major briefing came from Keating. In FitzGerald's mind the audit was simply to collect personal impressions of the issues of concern to those who chose to meet with him. Those issues included Patel conducting operations outside his competence and that ICU patients were not being transferred properly. Miach took the opportunity to talk with FitzGerald about the catheter placement issue.

By this time Patel's litany of surgical errors included having performed unnecessary operations — such as the removal of a patient's bowel on account of a suspected cancer, which was later found to be benign; the removal of the wrong organ; and failure to adhere to accepted standards and procedures for wound closure, often resulting in burst abdomens and incisional hernias.

In Hoffman's view, FitzGerald's audit was not inspiring any confidence in her that something would be done about Patel. When FitzGerald asked her what she thought should happen, Hoffman said that Patel should be stood down pending an investigation, but he allegedly responded that it was better for the hospital to have a bad surgeon than no surgeon at all.

FitzGerald did, however, discover an aspect about Patel's clinical patient notes that he found quite strange. He noted that, while it was not uncommon to come across medical records that are incomplete or inadequate, Patel's notes were in fact very well written but they didn't actually agree with the information being received from other medical staff.

The interviews for the audit concluded at Bundaberg without FitzGerald making any firm judgment on Patel's competence but did result in Patel agreeing to cease performing complicated operations and ensure that patients were transferred appropriately. FitzGerald returned to Brisbane to draft his formal report.

Hoffman had been increasingly concerned that no action had yet been taken since her last letter to Leck some four months ago. Having watched FitzGerald arrive and leave with nothing better offered than 'a bad surgeon is better than no surgeon', Hoffman was well aware that the audit had really only been a general review of procedures, not the full clinical investigation she had hoped for. She returned to the ICU to face Patel again, who now bragged that his employment contract had been extended to help the hospital meet its elective surgery target. It was the last straw. Hoffman was going outside the health system for action.

From the very beginning two years previously, Hoffman had been worried about Patel and had tried to get management to take notice of her concerns. Despite the lack of any action, she kept a meticulous record of each verbal and written complaint or observation she had made to her superiors. Sick of the desperate feelings she and fellow staff had about not being heard, she contacted her local Member of Parliament, Rob Messenger, who in a previous life had been a radio journalist for the national broadcaster, the ABC. Messenger was keenly aware that health was a pressing issue in the Bundaberg area. In 2004, he had campaigned heavily on a platform of better health services for Bundaberg and had become the main conduit for health complaints in the area. He also belonged to the opposition party in state parliament, the one not currently responsible for the health of Queensland citizens. Messenger could afford to run hard on issues critical of Queensland Health, indeed his political ambitions dictated that he do so.

Messenger already had a drawer of complaints from his constituents about problems at the hospital. He talked with Hoffman for two hours as well as receiving a copy of Hoffman's original letter to Leck outlining her concerns.

Messenger immediately sought corroboration and phoned Dr Martin Strahan, the previous Director of Medicine at the hospital.

Strahan let Messenger know in no uncertain terms that the local medical community was well aware of Patel's suspect medical skills and were all hoping that he would leave at the end of his contract. Messenger decided the issue with Patel was worth pursuing on the floor of parliament. If nothing else, it would at least be food for the ever hungry political journalists hunting news stories.

On 22 March, Messenger tabled the Hoffman letter in parliament and arranged for his colleague, Shadow Health Minister Stuart Copeland, to ask a question without notice of Gordon Nuttall, the Minister for Health. Nuttall was asked if the findings of FitzGerald's visit to the hospital would be released. Caught on the hop without any briefing notes, Nuttall was obviously unaware of the matter and told parliament he would make inquiries. FitzGerald was quickly called in to brief the minister later that afternoon but restricted his presentation to Nuttall to the fact that Patel had been performing surgery above his level of competence but had now been told to cease doing so. Nuttall was able to make a statement to parliament the next day, explaining, among other things, that FitzGerald's clinical audit was still incomplete but when finalised it would be provided to the Director General of Queensland Health.

But the public storm had begun.

Astoundingly, the first casualties were the nurses at Bundaberg ICU who were called in en masse the day after Messenger spoke in parliament. Once they had assembled, a furious Leck strode in and gave them an admonishing lecture about the Queensland Health Code of Conduct and their appalling behaviour in undermining confidence in the hospital, before turning on his heels and abruptly leaving. The Code of Conduct stated that 'unauthorised' disclosure of information was an offence.

The next day, with the apparent approval of head office, Leck wrote a letter to the local paper, the *Bundaberg News Mail,* in support of Patel.

By 24 March, FitzGerald had completed his report for the Director General. He recommended a number of systematic changes including a credentialing system and an audit system. He compared the rates of complications for Bundaberg with those recorded nationally, and maintained that staff concerns fell into two groups — procedures conducted beyond the scope of the hospital, and the lack of good working relationships between staff. He also noted concern about increased rates of unplanned admission, complications and wound dehiscence. He made no mention of Patel by name and infrequent reference to him by office (i.e. the Director of Surgery).

FitzGerald's official report also ignored the startling statistics that showed high rates of surgery complications at Bundaberg Hospital. Almost all the references to the Director of Surgery were positive and concluded that the problems were generic rather than confined to Patel. It did mention the need to complete the implementation of credentialing but did not highlight the fact that Patel still had not been credentialed by the College of Surgeons. No attempt was made to address the very serious allegations raised by senior doctors and nurses. The report did not propose that Patel should cease operating or that his contract should not be renewed.

Yet, in contrast to this official departmental response, FitzGerald wrote personally to the Director General of Queensland Health a few days later, saying that there was evidence that Patel had a significantly higher complication rate than his peer group and had undertaken types of surgery beyond his skills and the capability of Bundaberg Hospital. Patel's judgment, FitzGerald said, was below the expected standard and recommended these matters be examined by the Medical Board to whom he had written. He also identified failure of systemic issues including the absence of credentialing and privileging (the process by which hospitals assess and confirm a doctor's stated education, personal background, licensing and prior affiliations so as to grant the privilege to perform medical procedures at the hospital), the slow and ineffective response of the Bundaberg executive to staff concerns and the need to have the hospital management implement safety and quality systems.

On 31 March 2005, Jayant Patel departed Australia for the US with a business-class airline ticket paid for by Queensland Health after serving at the hospital for 24 months, seeing over 1400 patients and performing over 1000 operations. He had formally resigned just after Messenger's question to parliament hit the papers. He took with him an appreciative letter from Darren Keating, thanking Patel for 'his sustained commitment, ongoing enthusiasm and strong work ethic'.

4

'He doesn't bother for others'

The town of Jamnagar, India, was established in the 15th century and sits just south of the Gulf of Kutch, in Gujarat State. It is known mainly for a colourful tie-dye traditional cloth called bandhini. The Jamnagar Bala Hanuman temple is listed in the *Guinness Book of World Records* for the continuous chanting of 'Shri Ram! Jai Ram!' since 1964 — the chanting of the prayer continued uninterrupted even during the 2001 earthquake.

Jamnagar is also the birthplace of Jayant Patel and the city where he spent both his school and university years. A world away from the sleepy Australian country town of Bundaberg, it is here where we next visited in 2006 in the pursuit of some reasoning behind Patel's destructive time in both the US and Australian health systems. What might have helped produce a personality so medically ambitious yet so callous to the care of patients?

The flight out to Jamnagar from teeming Mumbai takes less than an hour. In typical Indian fashion the flight is often 'pre-poned' — an Indian English term for a change in departure time that brings a flight forward rather than pushing it later, with the result that travellers must always arrive hours earlier than any quoted schedule if they are to make their flight. From the air, Jamnagar sits in a flat brown plain with patches of vivid green irrigated crops. The airport houses rows of parked Indian Air Force MIGs beside hardened bunkers. The 10 kilometre drive into town on a crowded minibus whizzes you past a snapshot of surviving rural village life — cow pats being dried for cooking fuel, goats and cows wandering freely along the road, various sized Hindu temples, and constant farming activity.

While the city itself is a touch less frenetic than many other industrialised Indian towns, it still confronts you with its roaring traffic, dust, blaring horns, crowded roadside food stalls, rows of unfinished concrete buildings and the now ubiquitous electronics shops and internet cafes. At its centre is Willingdon Crescent, a busy collection of arcades built by a local maharaja after a sojourn in Europe and displaying a grand mixture of European and Rajput architecture. Lakhota Lake, home to up to 75 different species of birds during the winter months, is a popular walking area for families in the evening. Parks surrounding the lake feature large stones set with brass plaques proudly displaying the names of various benefactors and reflecting the prestige able to be obtained from service to the community.

Prestige through service is a notion not unfamiliar to Jayant Patel. His great grandfather, a respected farmer, was President of the Jila Panchayat (district council), and his grandfather, Keshav, was Deputy Chief Minister of Saurashtra State (a part of Gujarat before India became a republic). Patel's father, Mukund Patel, was a wealthy oil mill owner. The family's ancestral home, Mukund Villa, is a large two-storey building that occupies a full block in the prestigious old temple area of the city. Mukund died before Jayant completed medical school and his mother, Mrudulaben, then 84, lived alone in the house until local publicity about Jayant drove her out to a neighbouring town. She was quoted in the Indian press when the story of his actions first broke back in Australia as saying:

I am proud that my family has 14 doctors — my children, grandchildren, nieces and nephews are all doctors. And Jayant is the best of them all … He is very brilliant. There has been some misunderstanding … I don't know about any case as I don't read the papers … After some years in the US, he shifted to Australia. Only last week, he moved back to the US.

Born in 1950, Patel seems to have had a happy and comfortable childhood. His father was reportedly a very religious man, successful in business but prone to arrogance. One of the stories told of the Patel family is of the great grandfather who, despite his high standing and wealth in the community, seems to have retained a sense of humility. One day, dressed in his traditional farmer's clothing, he came to visit his son. The young Mukund, in response to a query from a guest as to who the old man was, replied in earshot of his own grandfather that he was simply a servant. Overhearing the remark, the great grandfather declared, 'I am not his servant — he is from me.' If this story is to be believed, arrogance about one's status and trying to maintain a supercilious view of oneself at the expense of others seems to have been incorporated into Jayant Patel's sense of values early on in life.

Patel's classmates have mixed views about his scholastic talents and social skills. Arvind Kotecha, a general practitioner who studied in the same National High School from Year 8 through Year 11, says he was always very clever in his studies but 'he doesn't bother for others'. Kotecha noted that Patel came from a large and wealthy family and had only a few friends at school, but still lacked sympathy even to those friends. Another classmate was quoted in the local Indian press as saying that Patel was born rich, with a grandfather who was a political heavyweight, and exhibited a flamboyant image. Patel showed a strong competitive nature early on and several of his classmates note how he could not work in groups with his fellow students and instead stayed aloof and expressed the belief that he knew a lot more than them anyway. He aimed to pass all his exams with the highest score in the class. When he received lower grades than his contemporaries he was often seen to attack the achievers verbally, criticising them and attempting to devalue their contribution and worth, even resorting to hiding their books. His classmates do, however, agree that Patel was not all work and no play back then. He had a reputation as a bit of a womaniser.

Dr Mansurali Mumdani, a general surgeon now running a private hospital and clinic, completed his medical and surgical training alongside Patel for nine years. He thought Patel's 'basic surgery' was good, but that Patel himself was arrogant, autocratic and a 'showman'. Patel always had to be the best. He was not content just to be good. To Mumdani, Patel had the natural gift of impressing people but believed so much in his own superiority that he represented himself to patients as a god — yet a god without pity. Questioned on whether Patel had shown incompetence in surgery while training — for instance, not washing his hands — Mumdani says there is no evidence of his behaving in that way. Perhaps, he adds, in Australia, 'there was no one watching him'. When pressed to offer an explanation for why Patel would continue to carry out complicated operations in Australia despite being restricted in the US, Mumdani lifts his right arm in the air, his hand formed as if to grasp a handshake, and makes tremulous quivering movements — 'You see, it is the surgical craving.'

The government-run institution where Patel obtained his Bachelor of Medicine, Bachelor of Surgery (MBBS) degree in 1973 and Master's degree in Surgery in 1976 is MP Shah Medical College, one of over 80 medical colleges across India. The college held its Golden Jubilee celebrations in 2005 and, like many of the government medical schools in India where entry is based on merit in national exams, MP Shah has attracted many bright students over the years who have migrated to the US and the UK soon after graduation. Several of its graduates who remain in India have successful practices and even their own private hospitals.

Prior to our arrival in Jamnagar, we had corresponded with the Dean of the College, expressing our interest in the medical training provided to Patel. The Dean put us in contact with the Alumni

Committee and we were warmly welcomed and even invited to give a lecture.

A quick tour of the medical school and hospital highlighted the contrast of modern lecture theatres and teaching facilities with the poverty of patients attending a publicly-funded government hospital in India. The corridors leading from the medical school to the hospital were covered in brightly painted quotes from Gujarat State's most famous son, Mahatma Gandhi. The general hospital ward was filled with patients lying on rows of metal beds, many with relatives seated on the floor beside them. We were shown documents about the medical curricula, and newsletters that portrayed the careers of some of the more illustrious college graduates.

The audience for our lecture on 'Safety and Quality in Healthcare' comprised some Alumni Committee members, current academic staff and students. All listened courteously after which we received a gracious, if somewhat convoluted and grandiose, 'vote of thanks'.

Dr RT Mehta, Professor of Surgery when Patel was a student at MP Shah Medical College, acted as his mentor throughout the completion of his Master of Surgery. Now working in retirement as an honorary surgeon at a local charity hospital, he was shocked by the news reports about his former student that suddenly appeared in the Indian press. He found himself interrogated on the phone by a 'woman judge from Australia' and questioned by Indian journalists 'in a harsh way', as if they blamed him for what had happened. In an *Indian Express* interview, he is quoted as saying, 'Jayant was an extraordinary student. Just too brilliant.'

Mehta exudes a quiet and dignified demeanour and is somewhat bewildered by all the fuss and controversy. He maintains that Patel was a brilliant student, but acknowledges he took risks. This, he says, is perhaps why Patel's surgical outcomes seem so poor. Mehta also offers another reason for Patel's situation — he was a victim of someone who held a grudge, or possibly of a racial attack. It is an explanation heard a number of times while in India and still visible on Indian internet chat sites that discuss the Patel case — 'Australia is a very racist country' it is sometimes said.

Patel returned to Jamnagar and his old College numerous times after graduating and moving to the UK. Each time he gave an impressive lecture about his successes abroad. The last time was January 2003, just before he was being recruited for Australia. He gave a talk about the declining incidence of breast cancer in the US due to early detection, seemingly off the cuff without the aid of any slides or other visual aids. Patel also told his Indian colleagues that he was 'on deputation from the US' to set up a postgraduate liver surgery unit in Australia. Everyone was impressed.

Yet a future in medicine in India never appeared to be on the cards for Patel. Soon after completing his Master of Surgery he flew out of Jamnagar for Rochester, New York. Here he began his surgical residency in the University of Rochester General Surgery Residency Program in March 1978. A letter from the Professor of Surgery at the University of Rochester School of Medicine, J Raymond Hinshaw, stated that Patel's evaluations 'were highly complimentary and he was promoted in the program'. In September 1978, he was certified by the International Commission for Foreign Medical Graduates.

Hinshaw, himself a prominent and well-respected surgeon, was to become an important supporter of Patel in the years to come. That support was given despite indications that Patel was exhibiting problematic behaviour early in his surgical career. In 1981, despite a promising start and a promotion, Patel found himself dismissed from Rochester's residency program. Hinshaw kept Patel in paid employment by putting him on as his research assistant until Patel was able to secure another residency placement at the State University of New York (SUNY), Buffalo, where he completed his general surgery training. Patel was certified first as assistant surgical resident, then as chief surgical resident at Erie County Medical Center in Buffalo until June 1984. He later became assistant professor of surgery at SUNY Buffalo and the director of surgical education at Millard Fillmore Hospital.

By 1983, however, after an investigation and hearing, the New York State Department of Health Board for Professional Medical

Conduct charged Patel with fraudulently falsifying medical records to show that he had taken the history, conducted the physical examination, written the progress note and admission orders for five patients that he did not in fact examine before surgery. He was further charged with professional misconduct relating to two occasions when he was the first resident on call in one hospital while moonlighting in another. In one of these cases he was unavailable to insert the chest tube for a left pneumothorax, a relatively basic surgical procedure. A third charge of negligence and incompetence was laid based on these seven cases. A charge of 'moral unfitness to practise the profession' was also made, accusing him of wilfully harassing, abusing or intimidating a patient either physically or verbally in an effort to coerce her not to cooperate with the investigation against him.

The board found Patel guilty of professional misconduct, fined him $5000 and put him on three years probation. Later asked about the leniency of the reprimand by a *New York Times* journalist in 2005, Dr William C Heyden, who served on the hearing committee, was quoted as saying: 'It wasn't anything drastic. He hadn't done anything evil to anybody. He hadn't killed anybody or anything.'

In November 1988, the American Board of Surgery in Philadelphia, Pennsylvania, granted Patel certification to practise as a surgeon. But that was just a temporary job strategy. Patel's new practice was to be in Oregon.

With the backing of Hinshaw, Patel scored a position working for Kaiser Permanente Hospital in Portland as a general surgeon. The Oregon Medical Board, seemingly unaware of the misconduct finding in New York, duly registered Patel in 1989. He arrived at Kaiser Permanente with exemplary references including the one written by Hinshaw which ignored his documented history of negligence, incompetence and unprofessional conduct and instead told a story of Patel as a resident who showed 'technical and professional brilliance'. In Hinshaw's opinion, the New York proceedings against Patel had consisted of the 'harassment of a brilliant young surgeon' whom he would recommend 'without reservation'. Hinshaw could not believe that Patel would write a physical examination note without having first examined the patient.

Having moved his family across to Oregon, Patel soon began the cycle previously seen of receiving early acknowledgement for surgical excellence. In 1991 and in 1992 he was voted Teacher of the Year, and in 1995 was voted 'Distinguished Physician of the Year' by his fellow doctors, in part for being one of 'Kaiser's busiest surgeons performing the toughest operations, rebuilding colons and removing tumors'.

He was also causing problems for patients. He seemed to have developed an obsession for performing surgery on as many patients as he could find. Kaiser medical staff were later quoted as alleging that Patel would often turn up, even on his days off, and perform surgery on patients that were not even his responsibility. In some cases, surgery did not seem indicated. A string of problem cases had developed, eight of which led to malpractice or wrongful death lawsuits. An elderly patient bled to death after Patel severed an artery and a vein during pancreatic surgery. One young man was left impotent. An elderly woman lost a kidney and became incontinent. Between 1994 and 1998, Kaiser settled out of court five patient civil suits against Patel and reportedly paid out US$1.8 million in two of them.

Kaiser Permanente conducted a review of his surgical cases in 1998, resulting in a formal restriction to practise, which banned Patel from doing liver and pancreatic surgeries, and required him to seek second opinions in all complicated surgical cases. Kaiser also alerted the state health authorities.

The Oregon Board of Medical Examiners launched their own investigation of Patel's Kaiser Permanente cases, focusing its review on four surgical cases in which three patients died. The patients included a man aged 65 who died in 1994 after pancreatic surgery, a woman aged 83 who died in 1996 after pancreatic and colon surgery, and a man aged 67 who died in 1997 after liver surgery. All three patients had developed complications and were returned to surgery because of internal bleeding before their deaths. The fourth patient, a 59-year-old man, had to have additional surgery to correct a colostomy that, according to the board's findings, Patel had performed 'backwards'. In an Australian television program interview some years later, the former patient said, 'They had to rearrange my testicles to take skin off to fix the urethra, and it left me impotent.' Following the review, in September 2000, the Oregon Board of Medical Examiners extended Patel's surgical restriction to take in the entire state by way of a Stipulated Order which restated the conditions imposed by Kaiser.

In February 2001, Patel took a leave of absence from Kaiser Permanente, then submitted his resignation in June. Kaiser's medical group board was reportedly scheduled to discuss firing him the next day. Kaiser now states that all surgical outcomes in its hospitals are tracked by a computer system allowing instant access to comparative data. Medical staff can lodge complaints anonymously through a national hotline.

Patel returned to New York to resume practice, but received an order in April 2001 from the New York Board for Professional Medical Conduct that forced him to surrender his physician's licence. The board concluded that he could be criminally prosecuted for what he had done in Oregon. Rather than face prosecution, Patel gave up his licence.

Yet Patel was still able to command favourable letters of recommendation from six doctors at Kaiser. One of the doctors, Dr Bhawar Singh, Director of Anaesthesia, who stated that he was a colleague of 10 years and worked together with Patel weekly, described Patel as:

> Very good, very skilful surgeon; deliberate in decision making surgery; asked advice appropriately; would ask for opinions if necessary. Dealt well with emergencies in a controlled way. Actively involved in training junior surgical staff. To my knowledge patients held him in high esteem. Gets on with other doctors. Generally got along with nursing staff — a perfectionist so got upset if things not ready for him, e.g. equipment. However, was professional in manner. Very conscientious and hard working. Nothing of concern in his personal life. Suitable for general surgery job.

Another positive Kaiser Permanente reference hinted at some disagreements among surgical staff but overwhelmingly supported his professionalism:

> Extremely knowledgeable, above average interest in surgery. Sometimes took on complex cases handed to him by colleagues. Found it hard to say no. Worked together in busy surgical department. Extremely good natured guy. Handled routine emergencies well. Well regarded by patients — liked him. 'Can do' guy. Vast majority of colleagues liked and appreciated him. He had a falling out with a very few of the surgeons at Kaiser. Not aware of any problem with theatre staff. Hard working guy, wonderful colleague. I missed him when he left. Nothing in personal life of concern.

These glowing recommendations, in stark contrast to the surgical restrictions and negative professional conduct findings across two American states, helped ensure Patel's success in gaining his job at Bundaberg Hospital in Australia 18 months later.

5

A Sad Parade of Management Failures

Tony Morris QC, like many senior Brisbane lawyers, works from a spacious book and artwork lined office situated in a modern high-rise building at the centre of Brisbane just opposite the state's courts on George Street. Below, during work hours, the crowded footpath is often dotted with bewigged and gowned lawyers scampering back and forward with their legal entourages in tow. It is hard to miss that this is the seat of law for most Queenslanders.

Morris was the government's first pick for the public Bundaberg Hospital Commission of Inquiry two weeks after Queensland's daily newspaper, the *Courier-Mail*, revealed that Patel had already had his medical licence revoked by one US state and restricted by another. He is a tall athletic man with a powerful presence, a reputation for high intellect, and a passionate belief in social justice. His ability to identify the Queensland Government healthcare system's weaknesses with trenchant accuracy brought him both enemies and admirers from within professional and public circles.

When we visited Morris in 2006 he had maintained his passion about the incidents of over a year before. Dressed in a crisp, bright blue-striped shirt with white collar and cuffs, he stands out as one of the city's more stylish legal eagles. He is pleasant and courteous, using his words economically and succinctly. He volunteers that he is prominent and conservative in politics and that his inquiry was set up as a political counterbalance to the Queensland Health Systems Inquiry, an independent statewide review of the entire health department headed by Peter Forster, a consultant with wide experience in the review of government organisations both within Australia and internationally. The Forster Inquiry had begun soon after Patel's return to the US and was soon producing its own damaging list of healthcare failures.

Morris speaks easily and enthusiastically of 'heroes' in the Patel story, citing Toni Hoffman, who blew the whistle to her superiors, local politician Rob Messenger and the newspaper reporter Hedley Thomas. It is clear he is worried about such events being suppressed within a modern healthcare system attuned to avoiding public criticism at all costs, and wonders what would have happened without a politician and a journalist both operating independent of any higher organisational agenda. He remains suspicious of what he calls 'collective mutism' on the part of both government and the media where other interests may dominate.

Yet he avoids talk of retribution in the case of Patel. In response to a question about why some of the wrongdoers had not yet faced formal punishment, he says that retribution rarely accomplishes satisfaction, and that it is entirely different from bringing closure to the affair. The focus should instead be on trying to make sure that the events at Bundaberg are not repeated. He does, however, make the point that while two of the principal players in the Patel tragedy — Peter Leck, Queensland Health District Manager for Bundaberg, and Darren Keating, Queensland Health Director of Medical Services at Bundaberg — were likely to avoid formal charges over the events, they would probably never get a similar job, and so could not be seen as avoiding any consequences for the events surrounding Patel's time in Australia.

But Morris was not to have the satisfaction himself of seeing his inquiry through. His aggressive questioning of inquiry witnesses and public expression of empathy for victims and whistleblowers led just a scant three months after commencement of the inquiry in May 2005 to a successful and unprecedented Supreme Court application to remove him as Commissioner on the grounds of bias. The court action was brought by Leck and Keating.

Though Morris was removed as Commissioner before he could complete his work, the volumes of evidence he had collected were left intact and much of the $3 million of taxpayer funds spent by the inquiry helped retired judge Geoffrey Davies AO QC continue the process and only add another $1 million in costs before bringing down his conclusions in September 2005.

For Geoffrey Davies, a tall, distinguished man with a full head of grey hair and a quiet and precise manner, his take up of the inquiry after Morris was not something that he originally wanted, nor a duty he says he at all enjoyed, particularly in light of the finding of bias against the previous Commissioner. For our interview he wore a smart pinstripe suit with his Order of Australia badge neatly pinned on his left lapel. The award is testimony to his sense of civic duty. He had only recently retired from a satisfying legal career when he was repeatedly approached by none other than Queensland's Premier Peter Beattie to head the new inquiry. Beattie's entreaties eventually resonated with Davies and he completed the inquiry as a vitally important and specific task requiring his utmost concentration and effort to ensure a fair outcome.

He freely expressed sympathy for both Leck and Keating, whom he feels were not unique in their behaviour but rather compelled to act in the way they did because of the situation they found themselves in. Consequently, Davies was not surprised when his investigations unintendedly revealed other examples of poor medical performance within the Queensland healthcare system entirely separate to Patel and Bundaberg. For Davies, Queensland Health as an organisation typified a flawed funding system, an absence of local clinician involvement, insufficient community participation and a lack of procedures to deal with doctors who showed distinct and serious personality problems. Again, he did not see these issues as unique and believes most other Australian health jurisdictions may be similarly compromised.

Davies, although conducting an entirely different mode of inquiry to the colourful Tony Morris, nonetheless was lavish too with his praise for Toni Hoffman's whistleblowing efforts, noting on the record her courage and persistence.

Between them, Morris, Forster and Davies, with support from an army of researchers and investigators, revealed numerous errors and oversights by individuals as well as poor organisational structures and procedures within Queensland Health.

Among the most notable problems was that there was no Hospital Board staffed by local medical and management personnel overseeing the day-to-day functioning of the Bundaberg Hospital. Queensland Health operated the hospital remotely from Brisbane, exhibiting the epitome of absolute command and control and centralised bureaucracy, such that local accountability or governance had virtually ceased to exist. The people of Bundaberg had no official mechanism to ask themselves, 'How do we know that our hospital is safe for us and our families?' The lack of a board also ensured that there was no way to influence the hospital's spending when safety was at risk.

The circumstances under which Patel was appointed came under heavy fire from one inquiry in particular. The Davies Inquiry found it 'breathtaking' that the quality control measures of Queensland Health for the appointment of foreign trained doctors seemed to be almost entirely restricted to the work of a private consulting firm based in Sydney that earned 15 per cent of a doctor's first year salary package for each successful placement. No question was asked as to why a well-paid US surgeon was choosing to shift to a small regional Australian hospital and why he had been unemployed for the previous 15 months.

The staff of the Queensland Medical Board were unfamiliar with the format used by the Oregon Medical Board and did not recognise what 'public order on file — see attached' meant. They were used to dealing with Certificates of Good Standing as used by many registration authorities to assist in considering the fitness to practise of an applicant for registration. These certificates contain a clear statement that the registrant is in good standing and not subject to disciplinary action or investigation. Under the pressure of processing 233 Area of Need special-purpose applications in the three months during which Patel's application came in, they missed that the paperwork sent from Oregon was incomplete and did not include the 'public order' documents as should have been attached in both the faxed and posted copies. It was a vital piece of information that would have considerably affected any assessment of Patel's surgical skills.

The order as stated on the website of the Oregon Medical Board declared: 'an amended stipulated order was entered in 12 September 2000. The order restricted the licensee from performing surgeries involving the pancreas, liver resections and ileo-anal reconstructions.'

The lack of adequate assessment and supervision of surgeons at the hospital also stands out. In Australian hospitals, and indeed in most hospitals in the world, the fact that a person holds a medical qualification is not regarded as entitling that person to carry out all the procedures or activities offered by the hospital. Instead, hospitals impose restrictions on the treatment that their doctors are authorised to provide based on a number of factors. First, it may be that a practitioner's qualifications or experience are confined to a particular area in which they have considerable experience and knowledge. It may also be that another practitioner is already providing the service and there is little point in duplicating the provision. Third, the provision of a treatment may require specific resources in the hospital such as advanced intensive care facilities. Without these, the treatments could not be provided safely. Fourth, there is the consideration of how easily patients might be transferred to a specialist centre. In emergencies, this may be impossible and surgery is performed locally, but for elective conditions the patient is transferred to the specialist centre. Finally, procedures may be restricted as a result of knowledge about the doctor's competence. This competence assessment procedure normally occurs through the use of bodies such as a Credentialing and Privileging Committee comprised of a surgeon's peers. These committees check that the candidate has the correct qualifications and experience, then make recommendations about the scope of the doctor's practice to hospital management.

Despite an updated policy on credentialing and privileging being issued by Queensland Health in July 2002, the practice seems to have fallen into disuse by the time Patel arrived in Bundaberg the next year, allowing him to start work without any proper assessment. Keating, as medical director, failed to have any formal assessment made of Patel's skill despite the fact that there were more than sufficient surgeons in private practice at Bundaberg to form an adequate credentialing and privileging committee; and, in the unlikely event of each of those surgeons having declined an invitation to participate, it should not have proved insuperably difficult to involve a surgeon from Brisbane or another regional centre, whether in person or by means of a telephone conference call.

Yet the blame for Keating's blunder can be spread further. The Davies Inquiry found that Keating's training for his position was wholly inadequate, and stated that it was simply unthinkable that the second-in-charge and first medical officer of a facility employing some 850 people with a budget of $56 million and with enormous responsibilities for the Bundaberg district community should have so little preparation.

Not only did Patel receive no effective credentialing or privileging, he was also not supervised. Incredibly, upon arrival he immediately achieved the exact position that was meant to be acting in a supervisory role for him. The Medical Board of Queensland had registered Patel on the basis that he would be employed at Bundaberg Hospital as a Staff Medical Officer under supervision of a Director of Surgery. He was instead promoted to Director of Surgery and then permitted to do complex surgery well beyond the capacity of the hospital even in the hands of a capable surgeon. Even after staff complaints about his operating skills, there was inadequate investigation. Indeed in November 2004 Patel had been named 'Employee of the Month'.

The evidence as to how Patel came to hold the position of Director of Surgery is far from clear. Dr Kees Nydam admits that, in his then capacity as Acting Director of Medical Services, he appointed Patel to the Director of Surgery position when another overseas trained surgeon who was expected to fill the position appeared less qualified. In any event, Patel was immediately appointed to a position for which he had not applied. Nydham explained this appointment as being temporary, pending the appointment of a permanent Director of Surgery. Scant evidence exists to corroborate the proposition that Patel was appointed as Director of Surgery on a temporary basis. Nor was there any suggestion of a serious attempt — indeed, any attempt at all — to fill the 'temporary' position with a permanent Director of Surgery.

In his 24 months at the hospital, Patel's surgery and medical practice was the basis of over 20 complaints by staff or patients, beginning just six weeks after he started at the hospital and continuing until he ceased working. All of the patients' complaints were verified when examined by other surgeons. Whilst the complaints varied in their seriousness and the formality with which they were made, some of them were extremely grave. There was unequivocal evidence of surgical and management failures and there was unequivocal evidence of poor practice in Patel's assessment, clinical judgment, surgical technique, post-operative care and follow-up. Patel was later found responsible for at least 48 serious adverse outcomes resulting in 13 to 17 deaths over two years — a complication rate twice to 20 times normally expected in the Australian healthcare system.

Yet the Chief Health Officer of Queensland had audited Patel's work in February 2005 and found nothing worthy of any further investigation. It was left to Toni Hoffman to get action on Patel by going outside the public heath bureaucracy to Rob Messenger.

The sad parade of management failures highlighted by the public inquiries also included condemnation of an inappropriate use of the Area of Need registration which resulted in Patel being appointed as Director of Surgery. Acquiring this position directly on arrival without following the usual route of seeking specialist registration via assessment by the Royal Australasian College of Surgeons avoided scrutiny of Patel's professional conduct. Given the small size of the hospital and its staffing difficulties, once Patel began practising surgery he had no peers who could assess his clinical skill and competence.

But why was Patel given such a senior role?

The Davies Inquiry offered a description of how Leck, a career bureaucrat, and Keating both saw their role as running a goods and services business trading in hospital services. This was best typified by evidence given at the Morris Inquiry by Peter Miach, Director of Medicine at Bundaberg, who recalled an official meeting with Darren Keating where he was advised by Keating: 'Peter, you have to understand that this is a business', to which Miach replied, 'Well, that's where the problem is, you see. I think it's a hospital.'

Yet it was Keating's view that Queensland Health central office wanted its managers to have. Each year the hospital budget was fixed on the basis of the previous year, with an additional incentive payment based on the amount of elective non emergency surgery performed, including complex operations such as those required in cases of cancer. Until quite recent times, hospital funding had also provided for a small percentage reduction from the historically fixed budget on the assumption that improved efficiencies in the running of the 'business' would enable a reduction to be achieved. Patient care and safety was not their first concern.

There was also pressure for managers to maintain the budget. District managers had been sacked for exceeding their budgets and, without a local board of management representing the community to argue a case in support of exceeding a budget on the grounds of safety, there was little incentive to try to do so. Because the achievement of elective surgery targets was necessary to obtain maximum funding for the following year, there was considerable pressure also to achieve these targets. In this respect, Patel was a considerable asset to the hospital business. He was highly industrious and ran many general surgery operations. Without him, the hospital would not have been able to achieve its elective surgery target.

The Forster Inquiry also found that the department took a dismissive and authoritarian attitude to complainants and there was premature abandonment of the first audit of Patel's results. There were numerous tales of advice from doctors being treated with contempt.

Yet health bureaucrats in Australia's Westminster-based political system are ultimately beholden to their political masters who are voted in every three years, and Queensland's politicians did not escape blame for Patel either. Two government ministers were specifically named throughout the three inquiries. The government itself was accused of a culture of concealment. In one highlighted incident, although Queensland had an excellent set of hospital performance data, it was wheeled through the government's Cabinet office during the dead of night, resulting in it becoming legally declared 'Cabinet in confidence' and able to be kept from public view. There were further accusations of misleading reporting of elective surgical waiting lists with the revelation of the existence of two such lists — one for people waiting for surgery, and another (unofficial) one for people waiting to get on to the waiting list for surgery. It was widely publicised that the Queensland Government spent 14 per cent less per capita on health than the national average overall and 20 per cent less on hospitals.

The public inquiries also revealed the difficulties for healthcare management in a state the size and make-up of Queensland. It has the most decentralised population in Australia, with 48 per cent living outside major cities and the highest interstate migration of about 80,000 people a year. It also has the highest proportion of the population in older age groups — a demographic time bomb for healthcare also faced by other developed countries.

In Queensland there are huge medical workforce shortages. Between 1996 and 2001 the number of medical practitioners had fallen from 317 to 305 per 100,000 population, much lower than the national average of 357. This has led to significant dependence on overseas trained doctors. In 2005, 1760 doctors were working in Queensland on temporary visas. Half of all resident medical officers were trained abroad. Between 1997 and 2003 the proportion of British and Irish trained doctors (a medical education system closest to that of Australia's medical schools) fell from 70 per cent to 43 per cent. These doctors could historically be relied upon to perform pretty much straight off the plane without any additional training. But it is not true of graduates from many of the countries now providing over half of the state's medical workforce. There are language and cultural differences, as well as the fact that their educational training comes from medical schools that Australia's doctors are unfamiliar with and therefore require closer scrutiny. The workforce and demographic problems are not getting any better. Although Queensland has three new medical schools nearly doubling the output of graduates by 2010, the expected demographic changes in the state's population mean that the increase will not keep pace.

It is a scenario repeated in many other health jurisdictions, not just across Australia but in the US and UK and beyond. The challenge of managing thousands of dispersed staff working to provide best practice healthcare while still attempting to provide the sort of individualised, careful, compassionate medical treatment expected by patients is serious indeed. Yet most of the time it works. Modern healthcare continues to save countless more of the sick than it has victims and it is responsible for preventing the premature deaths of millions more.

The findings of the three inquiries prompted by the case of 'Dr Death' show that weaknesses can creep into a previously robust and functioning healthcare system in sad decline. They may only be exposed when a rare but identifiable creature enters its system — the seriously personality-disordered doctor.

6

The Self-Obsessed 'Super-Surgeon'

From the moment the wider public first saw and heard about Jayant Patel's behaviour, media reports focused on the fact that Patel seemed to treat his patients with callousness, yelling at them and their loved ones, yet was also described by others in glowing terms. It was this sort of reported erratic behaviour that led us to begin seriously examining the Bundaberg Hospital events as an example of something much more complicated than the highly sensational story that was being told around the nation's water coolers — an evil doctor on a killing and maiming rampage, immune to censure from his soulless bureaucratic superiors.

There is also obviously more to Patel's behaviour than the explanation suggested by noted Australian anthropologist and active web blogger, Roger Sandall, who claims that Patel was driven by his cultural heritage to not lose his standing in Indian society and thus would never admit any mistakes or lack of knowledge that would diminish his status.

Cultural differences are not enough to explain Patel's actions. From all reports, he is more than just vain and proud. Yet the water cooler gossip is exactly that, gossip. Patel has never been described as some evil homicidal maniac or a deeply disturbed serial killer. If he had displayed such attributes, it is likely that any of the four health jurisdictions he worked in would have suffered far greater impact and his behaviour would have come to the attention of authorities far earlier, perhaps even soon after graduating and entering the US. Instead, his distinct personality served to make it difficult for a comprehensive picture to emerge on what sort of doctor he really was. Each person who interacted with him took away only a portion of the story. And as he moved from one healthcare system to the next, bits of the story were strategically left behind or de-emphasised, so that others would be seen as more important.

But there were always signs.

An examination of Patel's reported behaviour over the years indicates elements of a personality already known to psychologists as capable of causing great harm to patients when found in a doctor — pathological narcissism. The prominent features of narcissistic personality are grandiosity, need for excessive amounts of praise and admiration, and lack of empathy.

Narcissism is often associated with socially observable behaviours such as aggression, self-aggrandisement and distorted self-presentation. The relationship histories of people with personality attributes of pathological narcissism show consistent disregard for and violation of the rights of others, lack of remorse for wrongdoing and lack of connectedness with the feelings of others. Individuals display persistent patterns of impulsivity, irritability, aggressiveness, irresponsibility, recklessness and deceitfulness. Some may engage in repeated unethical behaviour. In the case of physicians, this could show up as insurance fraud, Medicare fraud, over-prescribing and over-utilising drugs for personal gain. Research findings suggest that individuals with pathological narcissistic characteristics are indifferent to the possibility of punishment, and show no indications of fear when they are threatened. This may explain their apparent disregard for the consequences of their actions and lack of empathy for others' distress.

The pathologically narcissistic doctor displays a grandiose sense of self-importance and attitude of entitlement. They tend to be demanding, insisting on special status and treatment, and becoming easily enraged by perceived slights. They also can be preoccupied with fantasies of success, power and brilliance, and go to great lengths to sustain an image of perfection and personal invincibility, projecting that impression onto others whenever they can. They do not recognise or identify with others' feelings and instead are exploitative, taking advantage of others to achieve their own ends.

Yet amongst all this grandiose thinking there can be elements of vulnerability. Pathological narcissism can be the result of a person's unconscious belief that he or she is flawed in some way. In this case the person might defend themselves against all others in response to the internal recognition of their own defective nature. This defence usually takes the form of trying to control others' view of them by being intolerant, blaming and demanding. They wish others to see them as extraordinarily special. Although individuals with narcissistic personality are often capable and ambitious, it is difficult for them to work cooperatively with others or to maintain long-term achievements. Their professional lives show a history of conflict, disagreements with co-workers and inability to tolerate criticism. Their interpersonal relationships are often also similarly impaired because of their lack of empathy, sense of entitlement, exploitation of others and constant need for attention.

Arrogance and grandiosity displayed by people with narcissistic personality can also be a cover for lack of competence. They tend to greatly exaggerate their talents and to regard themselves as unique and superior to others. The term 'malignant narcissism' has been used to describe a dimension of antisocial behaviour that is closely linked to narcissistic personality. Malignant narcissism is characterised by a narcissistic personality, antisocial features, aggression and pathological grandiosity. This type of narcissism is depicted as an absence of conscience, a psychological need for power, and pathological sense of importance which can combine and lead to cruel exploitation and use of others.

Major features of these personality characteristics may be identi-fied in Jayant Patel's professional history and reported behaviour as has been documented across three public inquiries as well as from interviews with his own classmates from his early medical training.

1. Arrogance and grandiose self-importance

Patel seemingly constructed a grand sense of self from early on in his career. His classmates in India described him as arrogant and autocratic — a 'proudy man' who 'represents to the patients as God' and was obsessed with being the best. From his arrival in Bundaberg he found it easy to assume the role of an expert surgeon from America, using a grandiose belief that he would find no equal within Australia's medical system which he somehow had wrongly construed to be considerably inferior to that of the US. He would consistently refer to Australia as the 'third world', and say that by working at Bundaberg he was doing everyone a favour. He bragged that he didn't need the money he received in his pay packet; that it was a part of his religion to give something back to this part of the world, and that it was important for him to show everyone how to stop practising such a backward level of care for patients.

Visiting Medical Officer at Bundaberg Hospital and former Director of Medicine, Martin Strahan, concurs that Patel's very dominant and confident character allowed him to ride rough-shod over others' opinions, assuming a high-ground of superiority when no such position was true. When challenged about his notorious indifference to hand washing during patient treatment, that had led nurses to label him 'Dr E. Coli.', he fancifully replied: 'Doctors don't have germs.'

2. Preoccupation with fantasies of success, power and brilliance

Patel consistently represented himself as a super-surgeon, variously describing himself as a specialist in cancer, vascular, trauma, cardio-thoracic and paediatric surgery. Before moving to Bundaberg he once again visited his old medical school at Jamnagar for a lecture presentation, this time regaling his colleagues and old classmates with the fanciful news that he was 'on deputation to the Australian Government to set up a hepato-biliary centre'.

He was eager to let others into his fantasies, though not always careful to ensure they could be believed. Charge Nurse Toni Hoffman, in her statement to the Bundaberg Hospital Commission of Inquiry, talked about Patel's persona and how 'his whole bravado about things didn't match up'. As she describes it: 'One day he would say he had trained in the States and had 15 years as a trauma surgeon. The next day he would say he had 25 years as a cardiothoracic surgeon. Every day there was a different qualification.'

3. Great attempts to sustain an image of success and personal invincibility

Hoffman worked closely with Patel in many emergency operations and noted early that his narcissism and constant bragging was backed by personal strategies to reinforce his position. He would tell patients things such as 'You're so lucky that your son had this accident today when I'm here' and 'I've been a trauma specialist for 30 years', instilling in them a false sense of security in his surgical skills. He would also ensure he treated any colleagues or staff at the hospital well if he saw they could do something for him in return. Hoffman remembers Patel buying presents for secretaries and senior administrative staff from the executive (non-surgical) branch of the hospital: 'They just thought he was almost like a god and they never spoke to offend him.' To this day Hoffman contends there are a few at Bundaberg Hospital who still believe the whole Patel episode was a media 'beat-up'.

4. Need for excessive amounts of praise and admiration

Many of Patel's patients have reported their initially good reactions to Patel's bedside manner. In stark contrast to numerous prickly professional interactions with medical staff, he seems to have worked hard to cultivate the god-like adoration he constantly desired. Beryl Crosby, an early patient of Patel's who later played a key patient advocate role as President of the Bundaberg Patients Association and a tireless campaigner for justice and truth through the three public inquiries, talks of how he gained trust so convincingly: 'He said to me, "We cannot operate fully on the liver cancer but I'm going to buy you some time, and I will fight for you". So when I went under the anaesthetic, I had so much faith in him I actually told him that I loved him for caring about me. I think that's how a lot of patients felt.' Yet Beryl Crosby never actually had cancer. For six months, Patel would earnestly prepare her for death, then suddenly turn aggressive if she or her daughter would question any of the test findings.

Confidence in Patel's ability was cultivated particularly effectively with the young and impressionable medical students who came to Bundaberg on placements. Hoffman remembers that Patel always paid a lot of attention to them, spoke loudly and confidently. He spent a lot of time with them, talking to them and telling them tales of how he set up an entire trauma unit in the US. To the permanent staff, it always appeared that the students quickly learned to look up to Patel and were often in awe of him by the time they left.

Bundaberg surgeon James Gaffield told the Davies Inquiry that Patel constantly craved professional acknowledgement of his work and wanted people to think he was better than average. Gaffield saw him try to achieve this by taking on complex operations or aiming to complete simpler operations as quickly as possible, and move right on to another to achieve as many as possible in the time he had available. In Gaffield's words, Patel 'was not content with being average, he wanted to stand out'.

Yet Patel was careful about the people he chose to seek admiration from. Those whose opinions did not matter to him, especially amongst the nursing staff, were lucky just to be ignored. Junior medical staff who praised his care, enthusiasm and generosity as a teacher confirmed Patel's self-image of a respected teacher, but any who had the temerity to question his judgment or ability were swatted away like insects. Thus he surrounded himself with sycophants and flatterers when he could find them and was otherwise content to work with people who had the good sense to keep their opinions to themselves.

5. Lack of empathy and a callous indifference to others' distress and suffering

As his classmates so easily recalled, Patel appeared unsympathetic to others' needs from his earliest days. He was good at his studies, but he didn't show much sympathy to even his own school friends. At Bundaberg his apparent cruel indifference to the pain and suffering of his patients was witnessed both in and out of surgery. Dr Miach, the Director of Medicine at the hospital, gave evidence about a procedure performed by Patel on a patient who wasn't properly anaesthetised. As Patel continued to operate, the patient began moaning and moving then eventually screaming in pain.

In the sad case of Des Bramich, who arrived at the hospital severely injured, arrangements that had been made to transfer him to a large hospital with appropriate facilities in Brisbane were suddenly blocked by Patel, with the declaration: 'I've been a cardiothoracic surgeon for 15 to 20 years, and if he needs anything I can do it here.' He then spoke to Bramich's wife and child in conflicting terms about how Bramich was not bad enough to be transferred to Brisbane but he would die without Patel's expertise. Patel began treatment only to leave soon after to perform a botched colonoscopy on another patient where he perforated the bowel and left the struggling anaesthetist to deal with the outcome. Returning to Bramich he proceeded to perform a pericardiocentesis (removing fluid from around the heart) despite no indications that the procedure was necessary. In doing so he used a 'violent stabbing motion' into the man's heart 'around fifty times' with a hard needle when the usual treatment procedure would be the careful insertion of a small bore needle. Bramich died. Hoffman noted in her report of the incident: 'Dr Patel screamed at the patient's wife not to cry.'

6. Irritability, aggressiveness, narcissistic rage, quick temper

Patel's history of abusive behaviour did not, however, start at Bundaberg. Journalists Don Colburn and Susan Goldsmith, in an article in the US *Oregonian* in 2005, reported that in the 1984 document filed by the New York authorities, Patel was accused of 'harassing, abusing or intimidating patients either physically or verbally'.

Beryl Crosby recalls that Patel would quickly become enraged when he was found to make a mistake. He yelled at Crosby and her daughter in the middle of a busy hallway next to the hospital cafeteria when he thought she'd failed to keep an appointment for a biopsy result. In fact his staff had cancelled the appointment some time before and after failing to hear from them with a new time Crosby had gone to the hospital to find out what was going on. When she finally located Patel in the hospital she suddenly was subjected to a stream of abuse for not keeping the appointment, despite explaining it was not her fault. In the midst of his tirade he also told her, 'Well, anyway, I can now tell you it isn't cancer.' It was a hard way for Crosby to discover that she had spent six months of her life believing she was dying.

And it wasn't just patients who were the targets. Glennis Goodman had been Director of Nursing at Bundaberg Base Hospital for 25 years until October 2003 and clearly recalls Patel's demeaning and abusive manner with the nursing staff in the short time before she left soon after Patel's arrival: 'He would just explode and it wouldn't matter if there were patients sitting there or other staff; he would scream at people. He had a very violent temper.'

7. Conflict with co-workers

With Patel's obvious intimidation of staff it was not surprising he had conflicts with numerous colleagues. Goodman noticed, though, that while he reacted scathingly to any attempt by her to challenge him on an issue, he remained quieter if there were hospital executives in earshot. Toni Hoffman's experience was similar: 'He couldn't take any criticism. When I confronted him, he didn't speak to me for the next two years. He would talk about me, in front of me, to the other doctors, but he wouldn't speak to me. That was an interesting situation.'

Patel's behaviour prior to arriving in Australia apparently wasn't much better. One well reported case involved second year resident doctor Sally Ehlers who spent a number of years trying to raise concerns about Patel's medical cases while simultaneously trying to fend off apparently amorous advances. The eventual fallout from her three year residency with Patel was a scathing review of her performance by Patel, and a belated investigation by Kaiser Permanente into Patel's surgery leading to his resignation. In Ehler's mind, much of Patel's behaviour toward her was about displaying his superiority and attractiveness and ensuring she was aware of how he could help her career if she responded to him in the right way.

Soon after arriving in Bundaberg, Toni Hoffman passed onto the hospital's Human Resources department a sexual harassment complaint from a female registered ICU nurse who had been asked for her phone number by Patel while they were both attending to a patient and then received repeated unwanted calls. Far from keeping the matter confidential, another ICU nurse later reportedly told Hoffman that Patel loudly announced to the staff of ICU: 'You can't do anything in Australia without getting into trouble.' Hoffman maintains that it was in fact this concern about sexual harassment behaviour, and not his surgical incompetence, that convinced the management to encourage Patel's departure, although there is no publicly available evidence of this.

8. Consistent irresponsibility, recklessness and deceitfulness

As the litany of surgical errors and unprofessional conduct revealed through three inquiries shows, Patel's rogue behaviour while at Bundaberg Hospital was relentless. But so was his deceitfulness in hiding his mistakes.

Declaring on his application for employment at Bundaberg that his licence to practise had never been subject to suspension or cancellation allowed him to start practising there in the first place. And when the surgical errors began, he continued the same tactic as in

New York and Oregon — producing misleading patient reports and discharge summary forms. At Bundaberg he routinely neglected to use the term 'dehiscence' (meaning a previously stitched wound splits open) in patient reports on wound recovery, though that is exactly what had happened in several of the patients he operated on. He even attempted to enlist the aid of the very patients whom he had harmed. Crosby recalls one woman saying to her that when something went wrong after her operation, Patel behaved as if he especially cared about her, saying, 'Look I'm going to give you my personal number here at the hospital. Anytime, you tell them to page me, don't go to your GP. You call me and I'll deal with it.' It wasn't until later that Crosby realised this was Patel's way of hiding the mistake from the hospital authorities.

Even as the whole episode was unravelling and the media knocked on Patel's door at his Oregon home soon after returning, he was quick to lie. 'I'm not him, I'm his brother', he confidently snapped back to the reporter's face. While not the best of deceptive tactics, its sheer outrageousness was enough to distract the bemused reporter, allow Patel to retreat inside. He would not answer the door to journalists again.

9. Incapacity to experience guilt or to profit from experience, particularly punishment

Over the course of his career when Patel was found to be negligent and officially disciplined, he absolutely failed to alter his behaviour. The string of surgical errors reported from New York and Oregon read little different from those at Bundaberg. In 1984 Patel was accused of 'abandoning or neglecting a patient in need of immediate professional care'. His behaviour at Kaiser Permanente Hospital was described as beyond negligence and just plain wrong. Yet Patel obviously disagreed. He would not change. Indeed, on his arrival in Bundaberg after successfully hiding from his new employer his previous surgical malpractice history, he seemed to have been spurred on to greater effort. He immediately undertook operations for which the necessary skill had been adjudged by disciplinary authorities in the US to be lacking, seemingly as if to vindicate himself.

It was this aspect of Patel's character that was to prove most damaging — not his sub-optimal performance of routine surgery but his enthusiasm to make decisions to carry out surgery that was beyond his competence. Eight patients who died at Bundaberg Hospital had operations performed by Patel such as oesophagectomies and Whipple's procedures which, unknown to his colleagues and superiors, he was banned from performing in Oregon.

But Patel just wouldn't stop operating.

7

A Compulsion to Operate

While an extreme narcissistic personality accounts for much of Patel's professional behaviour since graduating from MP Shah Medical College, it does not immediately account for what appears to be a pathological compulsion to operate.

Why did Patel keep pushing far past the limits of his own skills? Surely the ample praise of his employers, the adoration of junior doctors, the excellent pay and the fancy house would be enough.

For Patel, more was needed. It was almost as if he was addicted to the physical act of surgery. Perhaps it provided so much pleasure for him that to refrain from the act was impossible. The more complicated the surgery, the bigger the high. Sandall describes Patel as 'a man with a barely controllable urge to cut and slash', driven by a psychopathically sadistic streak and given to body-snatching 'in his obsessive pursuit of human material for his knife'.

This portrayal, however, conjures up images of maniacal madness rather than the almost desperate bravado observed during Patel's most serious surgical challenges. Certainly he wanted and apparently needed to operate on patients as often as possible. Soon after arriving at Kaiser Permanente in the US, medical staff noticed that he would turn up at the hospital to perform surgery on his days off work. If none of his own patients were able to be scheduled for surgery, then he would find others that were not his responsibility. The medical staff questioned whether, in some cases, surgery was even required.

It was the same in Bundaberg. Patel operated on 867 patients over two years, many of them several times. Within two months of his appointment his desire to perform large numbers of operations, particularly complicated ones, was already apparent. Toni Hoffman noted that in June 2003: 'Dr Patel was wanting to do very complex and large scale surgeries which really didn't fit within our scope of practice.'

As in New York and Oregon, Patel was over-enthusiastic in finding patients that he believed would benefit from his surgical skills. It did not matter whether they were his patients or under the care of another physician. He didn't even bother to inform the other doctor before operating. After this had occurred one too many times for the liking of the Director of Medicine, Peter Maich, he privately ordered nursing staff never to allow Patel near his patients and if necessary to even hide them from Patel.

This compulsion doesn't appear quite as extreme as the 'cut and slash' Sandall suggests when it is remembered that psychiatry has a clearly diagnosable condition for such behaviour, termed 'piquerism' — the gaining of pleasure from cutting flesh or removing body parts. Robert Kaplan, an Australian forensic psychiatrist and author, also sees elements of such behaviour in Patel but rejects its application as a cause for Patel's behaviour, instead viewing Patel's compulsion as a deeper extension of a need for god-like power over life or death — the ultimate in narcissistic expression. In other words, an overwhelming belief in his own omniscience, unable to be dimmed by the carnage and death created by his own hands.

As superiority complexes go, that's pretty serious. It's also something that can match fairly well with the life of a surgeon. Though surgeons certainly aren't gods and nor should they ever be treated or regarded as such, nonetheless they are accorded a fair degree of praise in most communities, including Indian society — just the ticket for a budding narcissistic personality.

In taking up a medical career and specialising in surgery, Patel knew that he would be held in high regard. The image of the surgeon in theatre, holding the power of life and death in their hands, runs across cultures and throughout our everyday education and entertainment. From the wisecracking 'saints in surgical garb' of the groundbreaking 1970s movie and television series *M*A*S*H*, to the slickness of *Grey's Anatomy*'s 'dreamy' Dr Sheppard, popular culture lionises the cult of the surgeon. With the advent of the 'reality show', even real life surgeons become stars, such as those featured on the Beverley Hills plastic surgery saga *Dr 90210*.

The real surgeons, whose lives are usually much more mundane than those of their TV counterparts, help promote this image through their own professional competiveness which often defines their success by the types of surgery they perform — their skill with the knife. The act of performing surgery can become the all-encompassing part of their persona. The more specialised and complex the surgery undertaken, the more the surgeon feels ego satisfaction. In the surgeon's parlance, 'nothing heals like cold, hard steel'.

What greater boost then to Patel's grandiose ideas than to see himself as a highly successful super-specialist surgeon in a large and successful organisation such as Kaiser Permanente, providers of the leading non profit integrated health plan in America. When he resigned from Kaiser, it was not sufficient to say to his old classmates that he was merely going to Bundaberg as a surgeon, he had to tell them that he was going on deputation from the US Government to set up a national hepatobiliary centre.

So while Patel was boastful and devoted to presenting himself as one of the best, his continuous acts of surgery fed into an over-inflated ego, and strengthened his grandiose personal world of fantasy — his narcissistic personality all the time never allowing him to see or admit any evidence to the contrary.

An analysis of Patel's surgical cases while at Bundaberg further suggests that the nature of his compulsion was very much unrelated to others and instead was squarely concentrated on himself. Patel seemed to consider operations to be an end in themselves rather than a means of improving the patient's condition or alleviating suffering. He regularly misdiagnosed patients and omitted to accurately assess the patient's suitability for anaesthetic, which led to more frequent incidents of post-operative heart attack and post-operative respiratory compromise. Whereas good surgeons are often reluctant to operate, Patel seemed reluctant to consider any other treatment option.

The Davies Inquiry took evidence from surgeons who had reviewed a range of Patel's patients. Dr Geoffrey de Lacy provided examples of high infection rates; poor wound closure techniques; injuries to adjacent anatomical structures including the liver, spleen, rectum, bladder and ureter; removing the wrong organ; missing cancers; failing to remove cancers at the operation; and wound dehiscence. He gave as an example of Patel's out-of-date techniques a failure to use a cholangiogram in the course of removing the gall bladder by laparoscopic cholecystectomy (gall bladder removal). In de Lacy's view, the number of patients with anastomotic leaks was grossly excessive. (When a surgeon removes a segment of bowel and reunites what remains by joining the two ends of the gut tube, the procedure is called anastomosis.) He noted that Patel would often select inappropriate people for surgery, a behaviour entirely consistent with someone compelled to operate and unable to find a patient.

Patel's rough surgical technique, no doubt exacerbated by his willingness to speed through an operation and out into another one, resulted in some post-operative complications that de Lacy had never even seen before. In one case the patient ended up with a bowel obstruction from 20 stitches through loops of the small bowel from Patel's attempts at a simple hernia repair. Post-operative management in many of Patel's patients was particularly poor. He failed to recognise or treat major post-operative complications including haemorrhage following bowel surgery, bile leak following cholecystectomy, dehiscence (the splitting open of a previously stitched wound) after abdominal surgery, and cardio-respiratory failure. Patel's reluctance to refer patients to appropriate specialists ensured his continued failure to recognise the mistakes in his own operations. In de Lacy's assessment, while some of Patel's surgery was carried out with an adequate level of competence, much of Patel's routine surgery was performed to a standard which de Lacy considered 'terrible'.

Dr Barry O'Laughlin, Director of Surgery at the Royal Brisbane Hospital, saw 42 former Patel patients. Of these, 14 had received adequate care and simply needed reassurance, seven required remedial surgery and there were 20 patients who had a range of symptoms and complaints that required further investigation. In O'Laughlin's view, half the patients he saw received a standard of care that was less than would be expected from a competent surgeon. When asked if he would let Patel operate on them, Dr O'Laughlin said simply, 'No'. O'Laughlin also came to the conclusion that Patel did not exercise appropriate clinical judgment in deciding when operations would not be the best option for the patient.

A separate review of Patel's surgical cases was conducted under the order of the Director General of Queensland Health in April 2005. This review looked at cases where there has been an identified clinical outcome or where issues related to Patel's clinical practice had been raised, and was undertaken by Dr Peter Woodruff. The review confined its investigations to those patients who had died, who had been party to a complaint or who had been transferred to another institution. A total of 221 cases including 88 deaths met the criteria for review while it was acknowledged that there would undoubtedly be patients who had suffered adverse outcomes who were not reviewed. The review determined that there were 13 deaths in which an unacceptable level of care had been applied to which Patel had contributed. There were a further four deaths which an unacceptable level of care may have contributed to. In 31 surviving patients Patel's poor level of care had contributed to or may have contributed to an adverse outcome, with 23 of these patients suffered major complications.

In all there were 48 patients in which Patel contributed to or may have contributed to adverse outcomes out of a total of about 1000 surgical patients over the two years he worked at Bundaberg. Woodruff himself had no hesitation in saying that Patel's performance was incompetent and that his performance was far worse than average or what might be expected by chance. Of the 13 deaths, seven or eight had been described by Woodruff as having received 'outlandish treatment' and involved 'absolutely indefensible' processes. He further speculated that eight of the 13 deaths were related to procedures which Patel would have been prohibited from performing in Oregon, leading him to wonder if in Patel's mind he was trying to 'reassert that what he had been precluded from doing in Oregon he was in fact capable of doing and that he was in effect re-credentialing himself'.

Yet it was not just Patel himself who benefited from his compulsion to perform complex surgery.

Extreme narcissistic personalities can prosper in large unwieldy organisational structures such as non profit health bodies. While they will certainly lie and deceive their superiors, ensuring that collegiate networks of select junior members of the organisation see things their way, their aggressive surgical work ethic can provide in the short term a temporary 'win' for a hospital.

In the case of Patel, he was quick to ensnare the top management level at Bundaberg. Peter Leck as District Manager and Darren Keating as Director of Medical Services needed a high throughput of patients to help balance the budget. Patel made sure they knew just how much surgery he could perform. Patel reinforced this positive view of himself in subtle ways as well, often providing small gifts to the hospital executive secretaries, making them feel recognised and appreciated. And he was always willing to host dinners out of hours for visiting students and junior staff, where he could build on his surgical showmanship.

Soon the executive were unknowingly colluding with him in his thirst for challenging surgery. Early warnings appear to have been ignored as they clashed with the appealing and engaging picture Patel had painted of himself to his superiors. Instead of seriously investigating the warnings, they rewarded him. And why not? In the eyes of the hospital executive, Patel solved many of their problems. He was an energetic and hard worker capable of doing long hours in surgery uncomplainingly. More surgery meant more income for the hospital. That certainly helped balance a budget; but running an under resourced hospital also involves dealing with frequent staff shortages. If a surgeon rang on Thursday afternoon and said they were rostered on the weekend but were unable to make it, the Director of Medical Services had to find an answer. Patel could always be relied on to say 'No worries, I'll do it', no matter what hours he had already worked that week. That is a valuable find for any manager.

Patel's perceived value to the managers and colleagues with whom he worked in India, the US and Australia is revealed by the unending stream of fine references and glowing reports of his work that allowed him to pursue his compulsive operating. These reports came from people who felt they 'knew' him in the workplace. They show Patel's skill in hiding the pathology of his compulsion and instead making it seem a part of the normal repertoire of a dedicated and professional surgeon.

Patel was and is always highly plausible at times. Personality disordered individuals often are. It is said of Dr Patel that he could talk himself out of almost anything. Most people don't come across such a disordered person in their lifetime and so find it hard to recognise the deceit. It's a bit like getting conned by a professional criminal. People always say afterwards 'But he seemed so genuine' as they berate themselves for falling for it. The police are quick to point out that professional conmen are good at their work. They make sure their victims believe them. It is not a failure of the victim, but the skill of the predator.

J Raymond Hinshaw, a prominent surgeon in Rochester, New York, is one such individual who found it hard to reconcile Patel's medical malpractice with his own view of him, stating in a letter to the Oregon Board of Medical Examiners that 'Dr Patel showed technical and professional brilliance'. This letter was written on 29 November 1988, four years after Patel had been disciplined by the New York state board for 'negligence, incompetence and unprofessional conduct'. In another letter to the board in 1989, Hinshaw defended Patel, claiming that the proceedings against Patel consisted of the 'harassment of a brilliant young surgeon' whom he would recommend 'without reservation'. In that letter, Hinshaw expressed disbelief that Patel would write a physical examination record without having examined the patient: 'such behaviour on his part would seem so bizarre to me from having worked very closely with him.'

Even after he had been disciplined in Oregon, Patel received favourable letters of recommendation from other doctors. Two of the Bundaberg references for Patel were from Kaiser Permanente doctors who provided glowing reports, checked verbally by the recruitment company. Both responded to the question 'Would you hire the person again?' with 'Yes'. One report, from a colleague of 10 years who worked alongside Patel one or two times a week, described him as a skilful surgeon who was very conscientious and hard working; the other talked of his 'can do' attitude and an 'above average interest in surgery', particularly for complex cases.

Perhaps then it is not so surprising that the letter of support for Patel provided by Dr Darren Keating at the time of Patel's resignation from Bundaberg Hospital thanked Patel for his 'ongoing enthusiasm and strong work ethic'. Keating was later to say that the letter was just a standard sort of thing you write when someone leaves, but the fact that it refers to not the quality of Patel's work, but its quantity, is testimony again to Patel's success in pursuing his compulsion to operate without alerting others to its sometimes dangerous nature.

8

Getting Away With It

While Patel stayed in Oregon throughout 2005, riding out the growing international storm of outrage over his behaviour at Bundaberg and beyond, the Davies Inquiry back in Brisbane was quickly getting up to speed following the debacle of the dismissal of Tony Morris as the first inquiry head. Darren Keating, the author of Patel's final glowing reference and successful litigant in the removal of Morris, looked like he was having second thoughts. He now conceded that he was aware of perceptions among staff that Jayant Patel was 'arrogant, abrasive, rude and potentially abusive'.

But why had this admission taken so long to come out?

As the inquiry progressed, it became clear that Patel had worked very hard to ensure he got away with what he did. It wasn't the single failure of an individual or individuals to notice the mayhem he was causing, but rather the outcome of a motivated campaign of behaviour and strategy to deceive his supervisors, colleagues, students and patients. Patel's campaign began with the deliberate concealment of his chequered disciplinary history in the US, followed by the ongoing avoidance of any systematic scrutiny of his work. In this way he avoided the formal construction by management of a true profile of his surgical outcomes. In its place was hearsay — personal opinions from some nursing staff and junior doctors regarding habitual rudeness and suspect medical knowledge, contrasted with similarly personal and passionate statements about his skill and care from both senior staff and patients.

Yet Patel's deception was helped by serious defects that were identified by the inquiry in the process followed to find and appoint Patel to the Bundaberg Base hospital. In hindsight it is obvious that, had Patel's true medical history been known, it would probably have prevented his practising as a surgeon in Queensland, and most certainly would have prevented his being appointed as Director of Surgery at the hospital. Reasonably simple investigations and inquiries could have brought Patel's disciplinary history to light, virtually at any stage of the process: before he was registered by the Medical Board; before he was employed by Queensland Health; or before he was appointed as Director of Surgery at Bundaberg. Many facts could be obtained just by using the Google search engine with the words 'Jayant Patel'. One Bundaberg nurse, Michelle Hunter, gave evidence at the inquiry that she did just that — by the middle of 2004 she had misgivings about Patel, did a Google search, and found the practice restrictions in Oregon.

The fact that Patel lied about his previous employment in order to try and get a new job is not in itself, however, an earth shattering discovery. Most employers will tell you it is an all too common tactic. But it is one that can work quite well, especially in large busy organisations that often use third-party employment specialists to handle large volumes of placement work. In the case of Patel, Queensland Health used the Sydney-based company, Wavelength. Judge Davies was critical throughout the inquiry of Wavelength's procedures, saying they should have checked with Patel's last-known supervisor and that references provided should have been current. Had they done so, it is likely that others in Oregon might have drawn attention to the shortcomings that later became evident in

Bundaberg. According to Davies, Wavelength should also have noticed the difference between the two versions of Patel's CV, one of which did not reveal a period of 15 months unemployment. Finally, Wavelength should have noticed that there was a public order on file and followed it up, which would have revealed that the order restricted Patel from performing certain surgeries. It would also have made it clear that these restrictions were the result of a disciplinary investigation in which Patel admitted a violation of the Medical Practice Act. If further inquiries had been made, the full terms of the stipulated order would have been revealed.

Yet, remarkably, Queensland Health had already just narrowly escaped another lying doctor prior to the appointment of Patel. Victor Berg was employed as a resident medical officer at the Townsville Mental Health Unit between January 2000 and January 2001. In his CV, Berg stated that under his previous name of Tchekaline Victor Vladimirovich he had completed a combined medical degree and postgraduate qualification in psychiatry at the Voronezh State University in the former USSR. He claimed to have been awarded the degree of Doctor of Medicine in Psychiatry in May 1977 and to have been a lecturer at the Voronezh University between 1978 and 1982, when he was ordained as a priest in the Russian Orthodox Church, and subsequently made a bishop in 1986. For the next two years he claimed to have been imprisoned by the KGB, fled the USSR in 1992, and was granted refugee status in Australia in 1993. Dr John Allen, the Director of Integrated Mental Health Services at the Townsville Hospital, considering that Berg might be suitable for a vacancy, made inquiries of his referees on the Gold Coast where Berg had been assessed as a clinician, and appointed him. The Medical Board of Queensland gave Berg conditional registration for 12 months to undertake postgraduate training in Townsville.

Not long after Berg commenced his clinical duties, Allen began to develop concerns about his clinical practice and performance. He raised these with Berg who took several months sick leave, and the contract expired. Some months after leaving Townsville, Berg submitted his qualifications to the Australian Medical Council in an attempt to have his specialist qualifications recognised. The Australian Medical Council referred the application to the Royal Australian and New Zealand College of Psychiatrists for assessment that made inquiries of Voronezh State University. The Provost advised the college that the university had no record of a degree being awarded to Tchekaline Victor Vladimirovich and no-one of that name had been a member of staff. In fact Voronezh State University had no such educational program in 1977. The Provost asked for copies of Berg's certificates and pronounced them forgeries. In October 2001, the college wrote to the Australian Medical Council advising them of what it had discovered about Berg's qualifications, with a copy of the letter also sent to the Queensland Medical Board. It was, however, only 13 months later that Allen himself discovered his suspicions were correct when he heard about Berg's false qualifications when attending a college meeting in Melbourne.

Of course, it must be said that the practice of medicine does not have a comprehensive history of rigorous employment checking. Until the late 1990s, in most western health jurisdictions, surgical outcomes were not measured and analysed to pick out poor performance. It was possible for doctors to be struck off in one jurisdiction and seamlessly move to another. Frequently this move was made easier by glowing and incomplete references. In the extreme, the balance could even be tilted in favour of the poorly performing doctor and against any colleague who wanted to raise concerns about clinical outcomes. Providing incomplete references has long been seen as a traditional way of moving problem people on.

Having successfully concealed the fact that he had been legally prevented from carrying out complex operations in the US before arriving at Bundaberg, Patel's manipulative and ingratiating personality immediately began establishing his worth to superiors. He quickly won the trust and confidence of his colleagues and employer, gaining a reputation as a hard-working and valuable member of the medical staff. At the same time he treated with disdain and contempt anyone who questioned his judgment or ability. Both junior doctors and nurses described how he would refuse to speak to or acknowledge them, sometimes for months at a time, and in the face of compelling reasons for communication. He would constantly talk about himself loudly and in self-serving terms. A number of witnesses told the Davies Inquiry that Patel would inform other staff that he was highly valued by management because of the elective surgery targets and would on occasion threaten to resign if his views were not adopted. In short, Patel made it clear to people that if they challenged him he would visit retribution on them and in any case the challenge was unlikely to receive serious consideration by management. Kees Nydam, the acting director of Medical Services at the time, described Patel as having an 'alpha male' personality. Others characterised his general attitude in more colloquial terms — 'kiss up and kick down'.

He also made sure to work with very junior staff wherever possible, a tactic made easier by the fact that, at the time Patel arrived at Bundaberg, the hospital had lost all of its surgical registrars. When Leck complained to Patel that he needed to reinstitute medical teaching, Patel quickly said 'That's alright, I'll teach them.' The new doctors who arrived for training had little experience in surgery so would not have realised that the levels of complications among Patel's patients were abnormal.

The fact that Patel played such a teaching role with students again stemmed from his success in convincing others of his perceived superiority. The University of Queensland, the major trainer of doctors in the state and the third largest university in the country, was looking to appoint a Rural Co-ordinator for Surgery for their Medical School based in the Bundaberg area when Patel's name came up. The position had a starting salary of about $90,000 and Darren Keating was on the selection committee. Patel's competition was a surgeon in private practice. With strong backing from Keating, Patel got the job and an Associate Professorship title from the university, despite the fact that other surgeons holding academic appointments at Bundaberg with higher levels of academic achievement (including Peter Miach who has a PhD) were only granted senior lecturer positions.

There is evidence that this manipulation by Patel to keep superiors loyal and subordinates silenced had been previously applied back in the US. During the 2000 Oregon Medical Board's review of Patel's cases at Kaiser Permanente it was revealed that a young doctor serving in a residency program under Patel at nearby St Vincent's hospital, Sally Ehlers, had been worried about Patel's operating procedures as far back as 1992 but felt her job would be on the line if she raised any issues. It wasn't until 1996 after Patel had stopped overseeing residents that she felt comfortable enough to bring up at a weekly surgeons meeting a case from four years earlier where a patient had developed infections and other problems after his colon was removed by Patel for ulcerative colitis. The attending surgeons were evidently concerned enough at the case discussion on Patel's work for the chief of surgery at St Vincent's to start his own research into Patel's other surgical cases soon after.

Patel's experienced surgical colleagues at Bundaberg were of course also not as easy to deceive or intimidate, and so required a different tack. He tended to avoid where possible professional contact with other surgeons and, despite the expectation of the hospital director at the time, did not take the necessary steps to become a member of the Royal Australasian College of Surgeons and so obtain full specialist registration as a surgeon in Queensland. Had he done so it is very likely that his disciplinary history in the US would have come to light. His isolation from peers was enhanced by his bombastic manner at work, which saw most doctors avoid him socially. Patel rarely, if ever, sought the opinion of other specialists or referred patients to them and was more reluctant than other doctors to transfer patients to Brisbane. He resisted any collaborative approach to treatment and was frequently in conflict with anaesthetists, feeling at liberty to countermand the orders of anaesthetists during surgery even though his medical knowledge was seen as out of date. The result was that many of those with whom he worked most closely — surgeons, anaesthetists, junior medical staff, and directors — accepted him at face value. Dr Peter Miach, a highly qualified and respected nephrologist at Bundaberg, who ultimately became one of Patel's most strident critics, trusted Patel to work on his own patients for at least several months. Indeed Patel's medical colleagues in the US seemed also to have been taken in by his behaviour. He was voted Teacher of the Year for two years running at Kaiser Permanente and received a distinguished physician award in 1995.

Of course, one of the best tools Patel had at his disposal to ensure his continued ability to operate outside the bounds of his competence was his position as Director of Surgery. Patel was not subject to supervision, nor answerable to anyone for his clinical judgments and was free to perform any surgery he thought fit. For all intents and purposes, he was at the apex of the clinical hierarchy at Bundaberg.

When mistakes eventually occurred, Patel was also successful in lessening their analysis. It is the practice in many hospitals to refer cases of death or adverse outcome to special morbidity and mortality meetings, which are attended by doctors from the hospital, and sometimes also from outside the hospital. The cases are usually presented by a junior doctor and followed by a thorough discussion of what could have been done better. The Royal Australasian College of Surgeons requires its Fellows to participate regularly in such meetings. During Dr Patel's time, the meetings were still held but there is evidence that he subtly subverted them, shifting the focus away from analysis. Helped by the fact that overworked senior medical staff rarely attended, Patel would use the meetings to teach younger staff about a given topic rather than encouraging open discussion. The consequence was that many of Patel's surgical complications never came to the attention of senior staff.

This deception may have been helped by the claim heard repeatedly through the Davies Inquiry that Patel wrote falsified and self-serving clinical notes. Dr Geoff de Lacy, a surgeon practising privately in Bundaberg, told the inquiry that Patel's clinical notes were clearly set out to mislead the reader. There would be instances of wound infection, poor incisions and leaks, but no reference to them in the notes. Instead the notes would be sprinkled with stock phrases such as 'risks and complications of the operation explained'. Patients regularly told de Lacy that Patel had only seen them for one minute in the pre-operative consultation and that he had not examined them. The notes would often contain textbook descriptions of operations which de Lacy found to be inaccurate when he himself later operated on the same patient. In de Lacy's view, Patel's clinical notes were dishonest rather than merely slipshod and they showed a surgeon trying to cover himself. In the 47,000 pages of case notes for Patel's patients there was not one letter from Patel to any other doctor.

Yet, even with this effort by Patel to hide his mistakes, complaints to management were still made — 20 in all over two years. How did these go unheeded? 'Complacency at best' by the supervising body was the allegation heard at the inquiry.

Judge Davies himself concluded, though, that while some of Patel's unchecked behaviour could be partly attributed to a lack of adequate administrative systems within the hospital, it could not account for the failure to act on the complaints. At the very best, Keating and Leck 'demonstrated a woeful ignorance of clinical outcomes at the hospital and a disconnection from staff'. He further speculated that under the administration of Keating and Leck the Bundaberg Base Hospital was much more fiscally driven and Patel seemed much more adept at meeting surgery targets which directly related to budgetary performance.

Davies was also critical of the audit at Bundaberg by Gerry FitzGerald. Leck had asked for an investigation to ascertain whether there was any substance to the serious allegations about Patel that he was receiving. It seems reasonable that after interviewing key staff members at the hospital, viewing a bundle of complaints, and hearing Hoffman's view that Patel should be stood down pending a full investigation that FitzGerald would have found something for Leck to act on. Instead, FitzGerald tended to focus only on the activities within the Intensive Care Unit and adopted a style of investigation which would, in Davies words, 'accentuate the positives'.

Political considerations in Brisbane taking priority over the clinical interests of patients in Bundaberg may have been behind this. FitzGerald, it must be remembered, was also by virtue of his position as Chief Medical Officer for Queensland Health a member of the state Medical Board. He was reportedly informed during his visit to Bundaberg that Patel had not been credentialed, yet he did not check the background to Patel's registration. If he had looked, he would have found a striking anomaly for a practising surgeon — Patel was not recognised as a specialist in Queensland, and yet was practising in an unsupervised position, without any peer review, as the Director of Surgery. FitzGerald was also made aware that the hospital was offering Patel a three months extension to his contract. The end result of the audit was a decision to have Patel restrict himself from more complicated operations but he was to remain in his position, as it was viewed by Brisbane as best for the hospital.

Certainly, Patel himself earnestly believed that he was important to the 'powers that be' at Bundaberg — Keating and Leck. The sources of such belief are not difficult to identify. Patel was indeed a 'money spinner' for the hospital. He performed teaching duties for The University of Queensland amongst interns and junior medical staff, which resulted in significant funds being paid directly into Bundaberg Hospital's coffers. The amount of surgery he performed not only improved the hospital's statistical track record, it also entitled the hospital to receive extra funding from Queensland Health. Moreover, based on the system of 'weighted separations' used by Queensland Health to assess such entitlements, the pecuniary value of his efforts was increased in proportion to the complexity of the surgery undertaken and the patient's underlying state of health. It is no exaggeration to say that, for each patient on whom Patel performed an operation which he was banned from performing in

Oregon, thousands of dollars flowed to Bundaberg Hospital regardless of whether the patient lived or died. The hospital funding system clearly made Patel financially valuable.

Forster's Queensland Public Hospitals Commission of Inquiry, which followed the Patel revelations, also pointed out that Patel came cheap to begin with. A Director of Surgery would normally be a registered specialist surgeon with Australian specialist qualifications, requiring a more generous pay packet. If they came from overseas and had been able to satisfy the Royal Australasian College of Surgeons that their qualifications and experience were sufficient for specialist registration, they would also likely have been looking at a higher rate of pay.

Tragically, Patel's monetary value to the hospital was unrelated to his competence as a surgeon, the quality of the surgery that he performed, or the outcomes for patients. Patel was directly rewarded for the quantity and complexity of the surgery performed by him, regardless of the good or harm done. Whilst his rewards were not a monetary compensation of the level that might be achieved in a large teaching hospital in an eastern capital of Australia or back in the US, they took a form which was possibly more important to him. He was rewarded with praise, with respect, with admiration. There could have been no more attractive 'remuneration package' for a man who seemed to come to Bundaberg with the object not of healing patients, but of healing his own wounded pride.

9

A Quality of Care Somewhat Lacking

The Queensland Government Department of Health, like so many departments in government these days, follows a 'corporate' model of presentation to the public. It has a snazzy logo, a simplified name (Queensland Health) and a significant public relations and advertising department. Its corporate headquarters, known colloquially by the inner city street in which it stands as 'Charlotte Street', rises some 20 floors up from behind a three-storey heritage-listed nineteenth century structure which acts as a glorified portico entrance. The former Walter Reid Building was a fancy brick warehouse elaborately rendered in Classic Revival style with Roman columns, large arches and burgundy-red windows. Following partial demolition after a fire, it was adapted by the government to serve as an impressive street facade for state offices. Two wide entrances into which lorries once passed now afford an entry and exit into the secure underground car park and a covered pick up and drop off point for senior staff and visitors. There are gates, barriers and glass screens to traverse before arriving at a protected reception area.

It is from these offices that countless media releases emanate in response to activities, achievements and criticisms of the department. As the Patel case unfolded, it was the responsibility of Queensland Health to assure both the public and its own doctors and nurses that it was responding effectively to the issues being brought to light. The Davies Inquiry, however, found the department's quality of care somewhat lacking. It wasn't just that Queensland Health had taken two years to obtain a surgeon's review of Patel's work after receiving its first complaint in May 2003, it was the perceived culture of concealment involving both the department and government ministers after Patel had left that bothered Judge Davies even more.

On 7 April 2005 the then Health Minister Gordon Nuttall and Dr Stephen Buckland visited Bundaberg in response to growing public concern. Staff were notified by e-mail that there was to be a 'staff forum' concerning the 'Patel matter'. More than 100 staff listened as Buckland announced that the outcome of Dr Gerry FitzGerald's February clinical audit of Patel would not be published because of the public release by Toni Hoffman of her letter of complaint to Leck. Buckland claimed that in the circumstances no decent doctor would now want to work in Bundaberg because of all this negative publicity. Nuttall reportedly urged staff to stop the 'rubbish' by voting out the opposition MP who had read Hoffman's letter to parliament, Rob Messenger. The purpose of the meeting was seen by many of the staff attending to be to discourage staff from raising complaints about clinical issues at the hospital.

Davies himself expressed the view that the main purpose of the meeting was to tell the staff that the audit report would not be released and to admonish them to move on. He did not accept Buckland's explanation at the inquiry that he was genuine in telling the staff the audit process had not been finalised and that it could not be released in Dr Patel's absence without a denial of 'natural justice'. The particularly 'unsavoury' part of Buckland's actions on that day stemmed, according to Davies, from the fact that Buckland well knew at the time that FitzGerald had reached firm views on Patel's competence, believing the complaints by staff were warranted and recommending that the matter be referred to the Queensland Medical Board. Later that same day, Leck was communicating with a zonal manager about the release of Hoffman's letter to the public and told him that the minister had told everyone that leaking confidential information including patient information was unacceptable and that whilst he supported freedom of speech in terms of raising matters with MPs, he would not tolerate the leaking of such information. Leck suggested that Queensland Health perhaps send up an audit team to Bundaberg to deliver some training sessions around the Code of Conduct and deliver some 'firm and scary message'.

It was this sort of evidence, beyond the perceived negligence at Bundaberg Hospital itself, that began to focus more public and political pressure on the government to widen the scope of its inquiries on the Patel case into Queensland Health itself. Davies had already started the ball rolling with the finding that failure by management to act on complaints about Patel was motivated by an unhealthy culture within Queensland Health to maintain their jobs above all else. Managers had fixed budgets. Fiscal considerations were a major focus, and there was a perception that staff had lost their jobs for failing to work within budgets. They were faced with a scenario that, despite pleas from senior Bundaberg doctors such as Nankivell for more resources, they could do little because they believed the corporate office would be unresponsive. Hospital managers were also required to work within a culture that was seriously averse to public discussion, at least to the extent that it could lead to publicity. Leck testified himself that they were required to make decisions according to a risk management matrix which rated significant statewide adverse publicity at the same level as loss of life. Loss of reputation of Queensland Health was equated with the loss of a patient's life.

With the Australian Medical Association (the peak body for doctors in Australia) led by its Queensland branch now wading into the debate, the call increased that the blame for Patel should not rest in Bundaberg but be taken to the highest corporate levels. The media was now full of reports on a whole range of health service problems, including waiting lists, clinical workforce shortages, the quality of clinical services, and the integrity of public reporting. Everyone soon knew that Queensland Government expenditure on health services was the lowest in Australia — 14 per cent less per capita than the national average on overall healthcare and 20 per cent less on hospitals.

An independent inquiry into Queensland Health systems was announced by the Premier, Peter Beattie, on 26 April 2005. The inquiry headed by Peter Forster of The Consultancy Bureau, specialists in private and public sector management consulting, was supported by a team from the Department of the Premier and Cabinet, Queensland Treasury, Queensland Police Service, Department of Public Works and Queensland Health. Two advisory panels of eminent clinicians and other professionals provided advice to the inquiry. Specific concerns raised by a range of professional groups related to Queensland Health's culture, excessive structural layers, decision-making processes, excessive numbers of administrative staff, bureaucratisation of clinical practice and care, and secrecy in dealing with information. Staff believed that this organisational culture had in turn led to bullying and intimidating behaviour exacerbated by a resource constrained environment.

Forster quickly established that many Queensland Health staff felt there was something wrong with the system in which they worked. The culture was described as an entrenched and negative one, featuring bullying, coercion and retribution on the one hand, and secrecy, evasion and avoiding responsibility on the other. In Toni Hoffman's eyes it was a really terrible organisation with endemic harassment. There were those who tried to do their best but the answer was to 'sweep the whole place completely clean and change the whole culture because the government is afraid of Queensland Health'.

The culture of secrecy and cover-up was perversely argued by some as entirely appropriate to protect patient rights rather than to avoid the release of information that was in the public interest. This secrecy is in direct contrast to the practice of *open disclosure* as used in many modern health systems. Open disclosure is defined as timely and accurate communication with patients and relatives following an adverse clinical incident or event. Research indicates that the use of open disclosure processes can significantly improve patient satisfaction. Failure to follow the practice often leads individuals to explore other avenues of redress through complaints mechanisms or through litigation. Open disclosure should come from a trained person with enough seniority to be able to raise issues with the hospital executive, who has been involved in the care of the patient, and who the patient and their family are comfortable with. The expression of the disclosure should include not only a factual explanation of what happened and the steps being taken to manage the event and prevent a recurrence, without implication of liability or blame for any individual, but also an expression of regret.

Many Queensland Health staff also reported to the Forster Inquiry examples of inaction or lack of appropriate and timely action by management in response to staff who were not performing or who were exhibiting unacceptable behaviour such as bullying. There was also a perception that poor performance was managed by transferring or promoting staff out of the problem. Yet even this procedure took too long, often 12 to 18 months, and there was a clearly perceived lack of expertise among managers in dealing with poor performance. Human resource personnel were also viewed negatively. The department's individual performance appraisal and development system was seen as next to useless. The official Code of Conduct within Queensland Health was viewed as being used mainly to threaten rather than to encourage staff. Written in an authoritarian manner, it emphasised formal prescriptive and bureaucratic aspects of the culture, rather than a patient-centred focus on care. In Patel's case, Leck reportedly invoked the code with nurses from the Bundaberg Hospital's Intensive Care Unit to squash dissent. The impact of this failure to manage staff properly included an unhappy workplace, low staff morale, high absenteeism and people on long-term stress leave.

The Forster Inquiry concluded that the department structure of Queensland Health did not support a responsive, integrated and efficient health system. Centralised decision-making stifled local initiative. There were bottlenecks in decision-making caused by the senior executive director of health services being responsible for 85 per cent of the department's resources. Some functions such as budgeting and media handling would be better delivered locally where the services were actually based. The number of levels in the organisation promoted fragmentation in policy, governance, service delivery and performance management, yet accountability and authority had not been devolved from the senior executive level. This centralisation further limited opportunities for engagement with local communities and other stakeholders. There was a clear need to change the organisation from centralised decision-making to clinician-led decision-making.

Forster recognised that redesigning business processes would improve responsiveness of services, including reducing waiting times for patients and reducing pressure on clinical staff. This would help achieve four main goals:

- to appoint and develop leaders who could inspire staff and develop the attitudes, culture and beliefs required
- to solve the workforce shortages
- to reduce adverse clinical events and to support clinicians in their efforts to continually improve clinical practices
- to improve organisational arrangements focusing on the requirements of frontline services.

In focusing on the wider delivery of services, the Forster Inquiry recognised the particular difficulties of rural and remote communities which are entitled to expect safe, timely healthcare. It recommended different models of care, more generalist workforce roles and improved transport assistance to provide sustainable services in these communities. The suggestion was made to work with local communities, other service providers, and education and training sectors, and to include competitive remuneration and incentive packages and ongoing professional support to aid recruitment and retention of a skilled clinical workforce.

Forster recommended that Queensland Health upgrade its risk management systems by establishing risk registers at all levels in the organisation (district, area and central office) and identify the individuals who are accountable for the management of those risks. Risk management systems are used to ensure safety and quality so that patients are not harmed while receiving care. This important aspect of patient care will be discussed in more detail later in this book.

Comprehensive reforms were recommended for a vastly improved clinical governance system in which the community could have confidence. The system would include: recruitment and selection processes; credentialing and privileging; incident monitoring and reporting; involvement of clinicians in enhancing practice; and comprehensive multidisciplinary clinical audits.

Forster was also critical of clinical governance procedures at Bundaberg and made several recommendations for Queensland Health. Clinical governance is defined as a framework for continuous quality improvement and is the system through which health services are accountable for continuously improving the quality of services and safeguarding high standards of care. This approach contrasts with the historical medical practice of the individual clinician being held accountable for the clinical outcomes of a patient including clinical risks. In Australia, following statistics showing in 1995 that 10.6 per cent of hospitalised patients experienced an adverse event, a large investment in quality and safety was made in the Australian healthcare agreement of 1998 to 2003. The Australian Council for Safety and Quality in Healthcare was established and functioned until 2006 when it was replaced by the Australian Commission for Safety and Quality in Healthcare.

Clinical governance requires the wholehearted support of clinicians who will expect a 'bottom up' approach supported at local level by training and resources. Performance targets and clinical indicators are best accepted if they have been developed using a consensus of clinicians. In the case of Patel, the Forster Inquiry concluded that Bundaberg Hospital's clinical governance had suffered a number of crucial failures including not identifying restrictions on Patel's registration in the US and the lack of proper processing or analysis of incident reports and events. It noted the absence of a morbidity and mortality committee and poor credentialing and privileging processes. Again, the hospital executive was seen as focused on the budget rather than clinical outcomes. Overall, the poor conditions of employment for doctors in Queensland Health were leading to a high proportion of overseas trained doctors appearing in Bundaberg and elsewhere.

The inquiry recommended an independent Health Commission to oversee the development and implementation of quality, safety and clinical practice standards throughout the state's public and private services and to monitor best practice clinical governance and patient safety. This new commission was duly set up and reported to a parliamentary committee, submitting an annual report on quality and safety to be tabled in parliament. Three directors were appointed with one responsible for existing Health Rights Commission functions including complaints, one responsible for oversight of safety and quality, and one responsible for arranging the recruitment of District Health Council members after a community consultation. This is designed to bring better public access to accurate information about quality and safety through reporting by the Health Commission to the district and area health councils. The health system outcomes are to be monitored on: health status and health determinants, patient outcomes, health service activity, expenditure and efficiency, workforce, the quality and safety of services, service responsiveness, and health service sustainability.

Clinicians across the state had expressed their desire throughout the Forster Inquiry to become more involved in decision-making for allocation and prioritisation of resources including using new funding to influence changes in clinical practice. Queensland Health had already developed some clinical collaboratives or networks over several years to focus on quality and safety, and to improve service planning and standards of practice in the areas of cardiac, renal and stroke. Clinical networks are now seen as a cornerstone of the new decision-making and leadership structure in Queensland Health. The idea is not new, with good evidence from Scotland, New Zealand and New South Wales that clinical networks improve decision-making and patient outcomes. Their structure within Queensland Health is expected to evolve over time and to acquire a unique local flavour. Clinical networks bring their own challenges such as the network interaction with the bureaucracy, when managers may seek unsuccessfully to control them. Indeed their success, as experience in Scotland has shown, depends on a 'hands off', facilitating style of management which was rare in Queensland Health. The patient-centric focus should assist in resolving any bureaucratic complexity.

The role of clinical networks is expected to empower clinicians by providing Queensland-wide clinical leadership in a specialty area to develop well-funded new services and better access while setting and monitoring clinical standards and training staff in the science of improvement. The work is clinician led; multidisciplinary; involves and integrates primary, secondary and tertiary services across a continuum; involves healthcare consumers; and explores innovative models of service delivery, education and staffing. Clinical networks are not expected to be involved in the day-to-day management of clinical services or be the employer of clinical staff. That is the responsibility of the area health services. The plans for funding allocations that come from the networks would then be given to health service districts to implement the plans and to incorporate the service growth into new or existing services.

While the Forster Inquiry clearly revealed the centralised domi-
nance of control in Queensland Health, it was reluctant to undermine some features of its corporate governance structure that it saw
as responsible for achieving substantial gains in 'efficiency and
accountability' over the previous 10 years. A number of submissions
to the inquiry had recommended the reintroduction of hospital
boards with authority and accountability for the running of individual hospitals as had operated in Queensland until 1992. These
boards can be viewed as akin to the standard corporation board in
the business world which exists to set strategic direction, focus
organisational objectives, appoint and manage the CEO, and oversee
governance including risk management. The inquiry, however, did
not believe that these functions were applicable to boards in health
services because the directions were set at federal and state government level. The decision has not won unanimous support. Glenys
Goodman, who worked at Bundaberg Hospital for a quarter of a
century, remembers the days when a local board made up of
respected members of the local community and a nurse who did not
work for the hospital formed an effective body to determine what
the growing Bundaberg city needed for its health care.

There were then 62 boards across the state and members were
politically appointed, although Goodman felt party politics played
only a small role. She remembers that it only cost $480,000 to run
all the boards in the state. Board members weren't paid that much
to serve. The boards were replaced with 16 regions at a reported
cost of $25 million. Carole Kennedy, formerly Assistant Director of
Nursing at Bundaberg, remembers how the money was found: 'they
took 2 per cent from all the hospital budgets for the first year and 1
per cent for the second'. In other words, the money was taken from
patient care.

Regionalisation was deeply unpopular in many rural health
centres. Goodman remembers that when the future Premier, Peter
Beattie, was Minister for Health, he toured the state consulting
people about regionalisation and almost everyone came out strongly

against it. But it went ahead, moving the whole state health structure first into regions and then into zones and centralising many administrative services in Queensland Health headquarters at Charlotte Street. The QH corporate office was born. Goodman remembers well: 'Once the boards were gone, I felt suddenly we were working for Brisbane all the time. We had lost our community. There were increasing numbers of bureaucrats turning up in Charlotte Street and it became impossible to fund staff locally.'

Forster's case against boards was curiously based on a number of major points which contrast with the successful operation of health structures in other Australian health jurisdictions. The first perceived obstacle was that the General Manager of the hospital was not an employee of the board and reported directly to the Director General of Queensland Health. This is not seen as any impediment in the state of Victoria where hospital managers are also subject to direction at the state level, yet even the smallest health units in Victoria such as Bush Nursing Stations have local boards of management. One of the key roles of the board is to appoint the general manager and set their strategic objectives. Forster also pointed to numerous reports of the inability of boards to properly understand the growing complexities of health service delivery, yet this assumes that such knowledge is inherently held by someone else — perhaps busy politicians or central managers already burdened with managing their own corporate budgets and staffing complexities. In Victoria it is assumed that training is needed for local health boards so that they are able to deal with their responsibilities. Two-day workshops cover governance, structure and function in legal frameworks, clinical governance, the changing face of the health system, strategy, risk management, agency strategy, finance and operation, board effectiveness, effective stakeholder engagement, ethical leadership and assessing the board's performance. The program was evaluated in 2006 and received high praise from the participants who found it not only useful training as health board members, but for many it was useful in their day-to-day business lives.

The matter of budgets as allocated by the Director General of Health was another concern about local health boards. Yet hospital budgets had never been a creation of the previous boards in Queensland but rather an allocation by the Director General, and boards focused on running hospitals, not on the broader range of community and population health services. This is similar to the approach used in Victoria and elsewhere — the funding for a local health service is set centrally but the way a budget is used is determined by the local board. It means that when funding is inadequate there is a mechanism for local people to express it through the chair of the health board. This would seem to be a process that would have helped Queensland hospital managers who were expected to keep within their budgets even when patient care services were suffering. In a system with a local board, when dispute arises between essentially the minister of health and the chair of that board, the minister has a choice between a political problem occurring if the chair resigns and goes to the media, or finding the funding to satisfy the local need.

The accusation also levelled against local health boards is that their members are outsiders to the health system, open to political influence or parochial attitudes that would act against the proper integration of public health services across Queensland. The Forster Inquiry supported this view from Queensland Health despite other jurisdictions having rarely seen any controversy about the politics of the appointees. Generally health ministers take advice on who would best serve the local community. Instead, it may be argued that it is a political bias that is keeping out local boards in Queensland. The Queensland Labor Party entered power in the early 1990s, determined to get rid of boards and has remained opposed to them despite failures in its own health reorganisation policies. Command and control seems to be deeply embedded in the DNA of the Labor Party and thus on into Charlotte Street. Under its command, District Health Councils are tasked with advising and recommending to district managers on the public sector health service needs of the district, planning for services and monitoring the work. These councils, described by many health workers as toothless tigers, also play a role in monitoring compliance with plans, budgets and the performance of district managers. A member of each District Health Council sits on the Area Health Council to provide advice to the general manager. It is certainly an attempt at localisation, but one still steeped in official bureaucracy and restrained by standardisation.

In the days of the local area health boards, Bundaberg Base Hospital board members had three things to consider as overarching concerns in their deliberations and communications:

- Is the hospital service being provided good enough for their own families?
- Are things being done the way they would do them in their own businesses?
- Do they feel assured that everything in the hospital is under control?

Given the decline in the hospital's surgical services just prior to Jayant Patel's arrival, it is hard to think such a board would have answered in the affirmative. Once Patel arrived and began practising, surely the alarm bells would have sounded strongly.

10

Rogue Doctors on the Loose

In an article published in *Annals of Internal Medicine* in January 2006, Lucian Leape and John Fromson, doctors from the Harvard School of Public Health and Harvard Medical School, Boston, Massachusetts, came to a bold and startling conclusion:

> When all conditions are considered, at least one third of all physicians will experience, at some time in their career, a period during which they have a condition that impairs their ability to practice medicine safely.

For a large modern hospital with a staff of 100 doctors, that translates to an average of one to two physicians per year. In medical terms these doctors will be considered by their colleagues to pose substantial threats to patient safety due to some sort of 'dyscompetency'. This is not a word you will find easily in any book of definitions, nor even most dictionaries, including even free online ones. It is, however, a term used widely within the medical profession when talking about an ongoing poor quality of care by medical practitioners that presents risks to the health of patients. The term first appeared in the research literature in the 1990s when sectors of the medical profession writing about poor medical outcomes saw a need for a new noun to 'describe the entire gamut of suboptimal behaviours — one that neither implies the cause of the problem nor suggests what should be done about it'. It seems that describing a trained and registered doctor whose performance threatens patient safety as 'incompetent' was not acceptable.

Today dyscompetency may be measured in different ways, such as by numbers of physicians disciplined by medical boards, complaints received by boards with respect to competency issues, or failure rates in recertification examinations. The prevalence of mental and physical illness, or substance abuse, is often estimated by surveys or referrals received by assistance programs for physicians.

Leape and Fromson's work said that the majority of dyscompetencies were due to impairments from substance abuse and illness. They were not therefore talking about the average dyscompetent doctor behaving like a Jayant Patel. Their research does, however, break new ground in attempting to quantify some of the more deadly aspects of modern healthcare and, despite acknowledged difficulties in estimating the extent of certain problems due to incomplete or vaguely defined statistics from many different medical jurisdictions, their research highlights the need for the acceptance of inevitable failures in clinical care. In exploring the range of problems encountered with dyscompetency (including mental and behavioural issues such as depression, substance abuse, personality disorders), they made a distinction between the *impaired physician* and the *disruptive physician.*

The impaired physician has a disability resulting from psychiatric illness, alcoholism, or drug dependence. The disruptive physician exhibits disruptive, intimidating or abusive behaviour that interferes with patient care or the process of delivering quality care. Examples of disruptive behaviour would include profane or disrespectful language, demeaning behaviour, sexual comments or innuendo, outbursts of anger, criticising hospital staff in front of patients or other staff, negative comments about another physician's care, boundary violations with staff or patients, inappropriate chart notes, and unethical or dishonest behaviour. Not surprisingly, disruptive behaviour by doctors has severe consequences for the health teams in which they are working. Harassed staff will experience increased levels of workplace stress, decreased morale, and may attempt to appease or avoid these physicians. The effectiveness of the entire health team is in jeopardy, and there is a greater chance of errors in clinical judgment and performance, and delays or mistakes in making and implementing medical decisions.

In Australia, the NSW Doctors' Mental Health Implementation Committee noted as far back as 1999 that there were consistent findings of increased stress, marital discord, alcoholism, opiate abuse, depression and death by suicide, accident and cirrhosis in the medical community. They also stated that the incidence of anxiety disorders, psychotic disorders, and even personality disorders, were likely to be at least as common within the medical community as within the general population. By 2004, it was reported that referrals to the New South Wales Impaired Registrants Program for psychiatric problems, generally mood disorders, had overtaken referrals for alcohol and drug misuse and accounted for about 80 per cent of referrals.

The incidence of disruptive behaviour by doctors is much more difficult to estimate. Surveys of nurses in the US suggest that almost all nurses have witnessed episodes of disruptive behaviour from a small number of physicians (4 per cent to 5 per cent) at their institutions, mostly verbal abuse. In May 2004, the American College of Physician Executives e-mailed a national survey to 7000 members. Nearly all of the 1627 physician executives who completed the survey had encountered one or more physicians with disruptive behaviour in the preceding year; about a third of respondents said they encountered problem behaviours monthly or weekly. Disruptive or abusive behaviours were most likely to occur when there was a conflict between the physician and a nurse or physician assistant, but staff were reluctant to complain about a physician's behaviour unless it was an obvious and serious violation of workplace rules. Yet even these survey results may be underestimating the full extent of the problem because they rely on voluntary participation. A culture of reluctance to report on medical colleagues often ensures low response rates for such research. It is also unlikely that disruptive behaviours are independent of other performance problems. For example, a physician who has alcohol or drug dependence or psychiatric problems would likely also display examples of disruptive behaviour.

While medical registration boards in the United Kingdom, Australia and North America have identified the adverse impact of physician abusive behaviour on patients and medical staff, personality disorders are often unrecognised. A 2004 report prepared on referrals to the New South Wales Medical Board noted that registrants with personality disorder often presented as 'disruptive' rather than impaired doctors. These disorders were difficult to manage 'when the registrant disagrees significantly with the board about the nature and attribution of the main concerns'. In an interview published in *Psychiatric News,* Dr Michael Gendel, a forensic psychiatrist who specialises in physicians' health in Canada, maintained that personality disorders were more common than mood disorders in physicians and more difficult to treat: 'There is a subgroup of people with severe narcissistic traits — who have little insight and take no responsibility for their actions.' In the same interview, Dr Michael Myers, Chair of the section on physician health of the Canadian Psychiatric Association, said that doctors who are perfectionists are often seen in certain specialties, such as surgery, that require extreme precision: 'If doctors are antisocial, it can lead to serious boundary violations and criminal behaviour.'

The Texas Medical Association states that there are three personality disorders that are most commonly found in physicians: obsessive-compulsive, narcissistic and antisocial. All tend to show histories of interpersonal relationships marked by conflict, exploitation of others, abusive behaviour, outbursts of anger and lack of impulse control. Both narcissistic and antisocial personality disorders are especially worrying within the health professions, particularly since doctors often hold legitimate powers of authority over those they are treating.

The antisocial personality disorder is commonly referred to as 'psychopathy' although this term is not currently in use by the two major psychiatric diagnostic systems used by western physicians — the *Diagnostic and Statistical Manual of Mental Disorders* (DSM) or the *International Classification of Disease* (ICD). The eminent psychologist and researcher renowned for his work on psychopathy, Robert Hare, describes psychopathy as: 'defined by a distinctive cluster of behaviours and inferred personality traits, most of which society views as pejorative'. These behaviours include lack of remorse or empathy, shallow emotions, manipulativeness, lying, egocentricity, glibness, low frustration tolerance, episodic relationships, parasitic lifestyle and persistent violation of norms. Hare notes that there are many successful individuals who have such traits, calling them:

> intraspecies predators who use charm, manipulation, intimation, and violence to control others and to satisfy their own selfish needs. Lacking in conscience and in feelings for others, they cold-bloodedly take what they want and do as they please, violating social norms and expectations without the slightest sense of guilt or regret.

Psychopaths have weak inhibitions for antisocial and violent behaviour, and they readily learn and adopt behaviour patterns that involve manipulation, deception and violence to attain their own needs. They easily rationalise their violence or deception as acceptable. Their predatory style leads them to exploit others and exert control as a means of proving themselves, using their positions to victimise people and enrich their own lives. They have a distorted sense of the potential consequences of their actions and, unresponsive to such consequences, their behaviour cannot be controlled by punishment, sanction or the fear of being caught. A 2006 issue of the *Journal of Forensic Sciences* (Yorker et al., 2006) featured a review of serial murders of patients by healthcare professionals over 36 years and found 90 criminal prosecutions from 20 countries with 40 per cent taking place in the US. Nursing personnel comprised 86 per cent of the healthcare providers prosecuted (a very interesting statistic in itself), physicians 12 per cent, and 2 per cent were allied health professionals. Over 300 patient deaths and 2000 suspicious patient deaths were attributed to the convicted healthcare professionals.

According to the Australian forensic psychiatrist Robert Kaplan, the medical profession 'has more serial killers than any other occupational group' — a startling claim indeed. Kaplan, however, attributes this to the fact that medical serial killers do not seek the usual goals of sex or money, but rather a power over life or death — surely the most potent of human emotional drives.

This is the realm of the most dangerous 'rogue' doctor — the sociopathic physician who is unprincipled, deceitful, unreliable, and capable of inflicting great harm and suffering on their patients over a prolonged period without being stopped.

Michael Swango is one such rogue surgeon who managed to fatally poison at least 30 of his patients and colleagues over the course of his career, before being caught and convicted in 2000 for three of the murders. As the press commented during the trial:

> The most shocking part of the story is that Swango was able to continue practicing even after he was convicted of the nonfatal poisoning by arsenic of co-workers in 1985. After being investigated for murder at Ohio State University Hospital, he still was able to find jobs as a hospital doctor in South Dakota, New York, Zimbabwe, and Saudi Arabia.

After serving in the US Marine Corps, where he received an honourable discharge in 1980, Swango entered medical school at Southern Illinois University when he was 26 years old. He was expelled after being caught cheating during an examination, but the school allowed him to graduate. Despite a poor recommendation from Southern Illinois University, in 1983 Swango got a surgical internship at Ohio State University. Soon after, nurses there began to notice an unusually high number of deaths among patients that Swango treated and suspected he was poisoning them by injecting paralysing drugs. The nurses reported their concerns to administrators, but were met with accusations of paranoia. The Ohio state hospital authorities conducted an investigation and Swango was cleared and allowed to retain his licence to practise medicine.

Swango resigned from Ohio State University Hospital in 1984, and began working as an emergency medical services technician at the Adams County Ambulance Service in Illinois. After Illinois police found arsenic and other poisons in his possession, he was arrested, and in August 1985 he was convicted of aggravated battery for poisoning co-workers and sentenced to five years in prison. Released in 1991, Swango re-established himself by forging several legal documents, including a fact sheet from the Illinois Department of Corrections that falsified his criminal record, and a 'Restoration of Civil Rights' letter from the Governor of Virginia. Despite his admission that he had been convicted of poisoning his co-workers, Swango was successful in his application for a residency program and began working at the Veterans Affairs Medical Center in Sioux Falls, South Dakota. In December 1992 he attempted to join the American Medical Association (AMA). They uncovered the poisoning conviction and informed the medical centre. Discharged from Sioux Falls, Swango managed to win a job as a psychiatry resident at the Northport Veterans Administration Medical Center affiliated with the State University of New York at Stony Brook School of Medicine. Learning that Swango had moved to New York, the Dean at the Medical Center in Sioux Falls informed the Dean at Stony Brook about Swango's history, and Swango was discharged. The residency director sent a warning about Swango to medical schools and teaching hospitals across the US.

In November 1994, Swango got a job at Mnene Hospital in Zimbabwe. A year later, he was arrested and charged with poisoning his patients. Swango escaped Zimbabwe before his trial date, and in March 1997, using a false resume, applied for a job at the Royal Hospital in Dharan, Saudi Arabia. A few months later, en route to Saudi Arabia from Africa, he was arrested by US federal authorities at O'Hare Airport in Chicago, Illinois. In July 2000, Swango pleaded guilty to fraud charges and killing three of his patients. He was sentenced to life imprisonment without the possibility of parole.

Yet while Michael Swango's psychopathy drove his serial killing, his career path and attitude reflected another important and related aspect of his personality — unremitting grandiosity — a sense that he was above the people he cared for. It is this same personality trait that surfaces in the case of Jayant Patel. They both considered themselves supermen and worked hard to maintain their cloaks of steel even while the law attempted to curtail their dangerous activities. Thus, significant patient harm and even death can be wrought by rogue surgeons who are not clearly psychopathic. And the implications of such rogues' deceitful behaviour in avoiding detection while moving hospitals is a major cause for concern in modern healthcare systems.

The cases of rogue doctors Richard Neale, an Englishman, and the Australian Graeme Reeves illustrate this challenge with chilling reality.

UK gynaecologist Richard Neale was found guilty by the General Medical Council (the disciplinary board for UK doctors) in 2000 of performing operations without consent, substandard surgery, unnecessary procedures, and failure to inform the general practitioners of his patients about complications resulting from surgery and other procedures. Neale faced 35 charges of clinical incompetence, professional negligence and extreme rudeness relating to his treatment of 13 female patients. His career showed a history of providing false information about his qualifications and previous medical misdemeanours. When confronted by patients concerned about complications and problems caused by his surgical work, Neale often flew into screaming rages against them.

Originally from North Yorkshire in England, Neale qualified as a doctor in London in 1970, and migrated to Canada in 1977 to work at the Prince George Hospital in British Columbia. On his CV, Neale claimed to be the Director of the North Yorkshire Women's Continence Centre, which had never existed. He also claimed to have been awarded the Royal College of Obstetricians and Gynaecologists Silver Jubilee Congress gold medal in 1988, an award he never received. At the Prince George Hospital, colleagues of Neale complained about abnormal levels of complications. Dr Eldon Lee, a senior gynaecologist who worked at the hospital, has described Neale as 'absolutely incompetent'. In 1978, Neale conducted surgery on a patient with benign tumours of the womb who was considered too dangerous to operate on because she had only one kidney. During the operation, Neale severed the kidney and the patient died the next day. He was banned from operating in British Columbia but simply moved on to another hospital in Toronto, Ontario, where in 1981 one of his patients, a 40-year-old mother of five who was pregnant with her sixth child, died after he administered ten times the dose of a drug used to induce birth. He was struck off the Ontario medical register in 1985. Returning to the UK, Neale successfully applied for work at the Friarage Hospital where he stayed for the next 10 years, reaching the post of director of the maternity unit before official concerns raised about his performance led to a reported £100,000 severance payout. Neale subsequently went on to work in Leicester, London and the Isle of Wight before the medical authorities finally caught up with him. At his sentencing it was reported that he pleaded with the council to accept his 'remarkable success rate' and blamed his downfall on two former patients who held a grudge — this despite more than 150 women eventually lodging complaints about his medical practices. The chair of the committee told Neale that: 'The evidence you gave to this committee shows that you still fail to accept responsibility for the circumstances which led to the loss of your licence to practise in Ontario Canada.'

Following the case of Richard Neale, the General Medical Council asked the UK Government for new powers to allow the council to prevent a doctor from practising in the UK on the basis of a judgment from an overseas regulatory body. These powers were subsequently granted.

Similar to the history of Patel, who had been before medical boards in New York and Oregon, but still had good references to secure a medical position in Queensland, Neale also passed from job to job because he had obtained references. One of those references was from Professor James Drife, who held the Chair of Obstetrics at Leeds. The General Medical Council held that Professor Drife's actions did not meet the standards expected of a medical practitioner and made Neale appear in a more favourable light. When asked about his reference letter for Neale, Professor Drife said: 'He told me he had been cautioned ... I didn't go into a lot of detail and I'm not sure at the time that I really understood the implications of the cautions.'

The case of Graeme Stephen Reeves, a surgeon working in the picturesque Bega Valley on the south-eastern coastline of New South Wales, quickly dubbed by a media already whipped to a frenzy by 'Doctor Death' as 'the Butcher of Bega', burst across newspapers and television screens in early 2008. Ironically, the Patel case had spurred increased efforts by the medical authorities into reducing the risks from doctors arriving from overseas, but Reeves is an Australian who had been practicing for nearly 30 years. Reeves was first investigated in 1997 by the New South Wales Medical Board's Professional Standards Committee after investigation of 14 obstetric complaints about his work at several northern Sydney hospitals. In one case, Reeves's treatment led to the death of a patient, in another the baby died, and in a third the patient's life was endangered. He was banned from obstetric practice, but moved to the southern region of the state and began work with the Greater Southern Area Health Service. Accusations continue to fly to this day amongst political and bureaucratic offices in the New South Wales Government on exactly how Reeves was able to continue to practise obstetrics at state hospitals after being banned. Some clues might be found in the fact that in the Bega Valley, as in Bundaberg with Patel a few years earlier, local doctors held the perception that the local hospitals were overloaded and under resourced, with the only alternative medical service involving a six-hour round trip to the city of Canberra. It has also been reported that at the time the area faced an acute shortage of obstetricians.

The Reeves case has been described by Lorraine Long of Medical Errors Action Group as the 'worst medical disaster in Australia'. Her organisation received over 500 complaints about Reeves mutilating or sexually abusing patients going as far back as 1999. The New South Wales Health Care Complaints Commission is said to have had only two complaints and not to have acted on them. In 2004 the Medical Board deregistered Reeves for three years for breaching the obstetric ban after it found he had lied his way into a position with the Southern Area Health Service. The Medical Board identified that he had 'personality and relationship problems and depression that detrimentally affects his mental capacity to practise medicine'. The report suggests that a narcissistic personality disorder may explain his 'arrogant contempt for the authority ... of the Medical Board'. Astonishingly, eight GPs had written to the board in support of Reeves. Subsequently they defended themselves by saying that he had been deregistered not for medical errors, but only for misrepresenting his working conditions (that he was banned from practicing obstetrics).

Just as Jayant Patel had evaded the medical regulatory authorities in New York, Oregon and Queensland, in part aided by references that were less than the whole truth, Richard Neale and Graeme Reeves had managed to keep doing what they wanted to do. When Professor Drife was brought before the General Medical Council about an inaccurate reference allowing Neale to hold three other posts before being caught, he was told:

> If you write a reference which is untrue, or you failed either deliberately to mention something which is material or negative, or you recklessly failed to turn your mind towards the fact that you should have, you are culpable as far as we are concerned ... you need to be clear about not only what you put into references, but what you *should* put into references.

Yet, as noted by the council, doctors are in part protected against the consequences of their unethical and even sociopathic behaviour by the medical training system and work culture itself: 'too often rogue doctors are protected by a code of silence among those who educate, train, and supervise them in the healthcare industry.'

In the face of this pessimism, Professor Sir Graeme Catto, a previous president of the UK General Medical Council, believes that the growing extent of international medical migration will lead eventually to 'medical passports' recognised by regulatory authorities around the world and containing all relevant information on a doctor's work history, including any restrictions, sanctions or deregistration. It is this system he believes that will severely curtail a rogue doctor's global rampage.

Whatever systems are used to try and find and stop rogue doctors, above all else health professionals need to be sure that their concerns about clinical standards will be openly and impartially investigated. Where it eventuates that the issue is poor professional performance, then successful policies must exist to deal with the matter appropriately. An outstanding feature of the case histories of most rogue doctors is that early concerns were not investigated to the satisfaction of the whistleblowers. Consequently, whistleblowers are forced to go outside the system, using the media, public protest or political lobbying to have their concerns properly investigated. Patel's case is a clear example of how such actions, while well-intended and indeed necessary, can erode confidence in an entire hospital, placing immense stress on staff, patients and families. This is not to blame the whistleblowers but to make the point that open, honest and timely investigation undertaken within an organisation avoids the potentially damaging aftermath — an aftermath which, paradoxically, can make people fearful of disclosing mistakes in the future. Unfortunately many modern health organisations are renowned for their gap between rhetoric and reality. Some may even have a long-standing culture of concealment, blame and scapegoating.

It is not surprising that many health professionals have little faith that anything will change. The change has to come from management establishing its honesty and open accountability, which leads to the trust and belief that things can change. Only with this approach we will have the chance to detect and stop the next rogue surgeon who enters our healthcare system.

11

It's All About Outcomes

> … comparing the mortality at a certain semi private hospital of over 200 beds with that of four of the best general hospitals in America, having a total of 1200 beds … clearly showed that the semi-private hospital did not only do more operations, but that the mortality was much lower, especially in some of the more difficult branches of surgery.

So wrote Dr Ernest Amory Codman in 1914. He went on to speculate about what factors might have produced such an apparently anomalous result — that a small hospital might have better outcomes than larger, more prestigious institutions. Among the facts he cited were the volume of operations, the skill of the surgeons, the medical condition of the patients, the financial condition of the hospitals, and the way in which surgical departments organised the placing of particular patients with particular surgeons during the process of triage. The phenomena he was describing we now know has profound implications for modern-day hospital and healthcare policy — the relationship between the volume of medical procedures performed and the outcomes of such procedures. This relationship has been shown to be a complex one. More operations does not in fact necessarily lead to better outcomes.

A graduate of the prestigious Harvard Medical School, Codman is often credited with the founding of what is today known as *outcomes management* in patient care. Codman is thought to be the first American doctor to follow the progress of patients through their entire treatment and recovery in a systematic manner, keeping track via 'End Result Cards' which contained basic demographic data on the patient, diagnosis, treatment and outcome. Each patient was followed up on for at least one year to observe long-term outcomes. The aim of this procedure was to establish a system that offered the chance to identify clinical misadventures, with the examination of such occurrences providing a basis for better future care of all patients. According to Codman:

> We believe it is the duty of every hospital to establish a follow-up system, so that as far as possible the result of every case will be available at all times for investigation by members of the staff, the trustees, or administration, or by other authorised investigators or statisticians.

Codman was also a fierce proponent of the provision of information gleaned from that outcomes management process to the wider public, believing that patients should be guided in their choices of physicians and hospitals by knowledge of previous treatment outcomes. His work anticipated many contemporary approaches in healthcare including quality monitoring and assurance, establishing accountability, and allocating and managing resources efficiently.

Yet even before Codman, the seeds of modern medical outcomes management can be clearly seen in the work of not a doctor, but that most celebrated of caring health professionals, Florence Nightingale. She is credited with undertaking one of the first ever clinical audits, an important process in outcomes management and defined today by the UK National Health service as 'a quality improvement process that seeks to improve patient care and outcomes through systematic review of care against explicit criteria and the implementation of change'.

It was during the bitter Crimean War of 1853–1856 in eastern Europe between the Russian Empire and the France–Britain–Sardinia–Nassau alliance that Florence Nightingale arrived at the Scutari army barracks in Turkey to find appallingly unsanitary conditions and a high mortality rate among injured or ill soldiers. She and her team of 38 nurses worked tirelessly in the face of overcrowding, a shortage of medicine, mass infections, poor nutrition and official indifference from Britain. Six months later the British Government finally sent supporting personnel and equipment and sanitary conditions at the barracks were vastly improved. The death rate began to fall and was duly noted by the methodical nurse. The well-educated daughter of an upper-class English family, Nightingale was already a keen enthusiast of science and the burgeoning use of statistics to describe cause and effect. She had been keeping meticulous records of the mortality rates among the hospital patients. When she eventually returned to England she was able to produce a series of statistical graphs and figures from her Crimean experience illustrating how the effects of improved hygiene and medical care affected mortality. These were instrumental in overcoming the resistance of the doctors and officers to Florence Nightingale's new nursing procedures. Her methodological approach, as well as the emphasis on uniformity and comparability of the results of health care, would sit well within any modern process of outcomes management.

Whilst Nightingale's 'epidemiological' audit is in contrast with Codman's more 'clinical' approach, these two methods serve as early examples of the different methodologies that can be used in the process of improving patient outcomes.

Yet sadly, despite the success of Nightingale and Codman, the clinical audit was slow to catch on. This situation was to remain for the next 130 or so years, with only a minority of healthcare staff embracing the process as a means of evaluating the quality of care delivered to patients. Today the clinical audit process is much more accepted and best viewed as a cycle within which there are stages that follow the systematic processes of establishing best practice; measuring against criteria; taking action to improve care; and monitoring to sustain improvement. As the process continues, each cycle aspires to a higher level of quality.

The first stage of any clinical audit involves the selection of a topic or issue to be audited, and is likely to involve measuring adherence to healthcare processes that have been shown to produce the best outcomes for patients. Selection of an audit topic is influenced by factors including national standards and guidelines; problem areas encountered in practice; recommendations from patients and the public; and areas of high volume, high risk or high cost, in which improvements can be made. Stage two defines explicit criteria for a measurable outcome of care and the threshold of the expected compliance for each criterion. Stage 3 involves the collection of data. Data may be collected from computerised information systems or manually, depending on the outcome being measured. In either case, considerations need to be given to what data will be collected, where the data will be found, and who will do the data collection. Stage four is the analysis stage, when the results of the data collection are compared with criteria and standards. The end stage of analysis is concluding how well the standards were met or identifying reasons why not. The final stage is all about implementing change. Once the results of the audit have been published and discussed, an agreement must be reached about the recommendations for change, preferably using an action plan to record these recommendations, who has agreed to do what and by when. Sustaining the effects of the clinical audit is encouraged by repeating it, with the re-audit ideally demonstrating that changes have been implemented and that improvements have been made. Further changes may then be required, leading to additional re-audits. Results of the audit would be disseminated both locally to participating staff and others, and through scientific journals.

With the growth of information derived from these audits of patient outcomes since the 1980s has come the establishment of research into the relationship between volume and outcome in the delivery of health services. The field is still relatively young, however, and that research has not always been of a consistent scientific standard. A systematic and rigorous review in 2002 from researchers at the Mount Sinai School of medicine in New York used a conceptual model that identified a series of critical factors that needed to be addressed to fully delineate the relationship between volume and quality of care. Of the 135 studies covering eight conditions and procedures that were examined in the review, only a minority of studies were considered of sufficient quality to give robust results. It was found that only 16 studies considered the independent effects of both physician and hospital volume. Twenty-four used clinical data to adjust for differences among patients in severity and comorbidity, but only four reported statistically robust models. Only four adjusted for differences in specific processes of care, and a mere two addressed appropriateness of patient selection.

Despite this lack of methodological rigour, the uniformity with which the published research expresses the existence of the association between volume and outcome is compelling. No study demonstrated a statistically significant association in the opposite direction. Yet many questions about the nature and causes of the association remain unanswered. Studies of the same procedure or condition typically employed widely varying definitions of high and low volume, precluding definitive conclusions about the nature of its relationship to outcome. We do not know, for example, whether a volume threshold exists above which outcomes do not continue to improve with further volume increases.

What we can be certain of is that in today's modern hospital an emphasis on safety and quality must include attention to volume and outcome measures that are up to date and accessible on an ongoing basis so that performance can be monitored and interventions applied when needed. The consequences of such an approach are particularly relevant for patients served by small rural and regional hospitals. In these areas there seems to be an unrelenting trend towards the centralisation of clinical services in the name of efficiency — whether economic or clinical. Yet the discussion about volume and outcome cannot be limited to an economic and clinical one. The needs of a local community should be taken into account and the balance struck between clinical outcomes and the community's needs. Hospitals are important sources of health employment, as well as jobs provided to those who provide ancillary services such as pharmacists, cleaners, tradespeople, newsagents and others.

Centralisation of clinical services inevitably results in iniquity for people living in rural areas, as already evidenced by recent research showing poorer outcomes for patients with cancer in rural Australia. Decisions need to be taken to determine how the volume of surgical procedures and treatments relate to an acceptable quality of care and where that care should be provided. For Bundaberg Hospital, the relationship between volume and outcomes was behind Charge Nurse Toni Hoffman's concerns about Jayant Patel's decision to go ahead with an oesophagectomy soon after arriving. Hoffman drew attention to the fact that Bundaberg was not staffed to undertake procedures of this complexity. The outcome for a specific procedure such as oesophagectomy depends on the volume that a hospital undertakes. The more oesophagectomies that an operating team does, the better the results they will get — 30 cases a year is regarded as a minimum.

Available research does not shed much light on what specific factors explain outcome differences between high- and low-volume medical providers. No longitudinal studies (and very few of any good design) address the important question of how much variability, especially among low-volume providers, is due to chance. Few investigations have assessed differences in specific clinical processes of care, especially those known to affect outcomes. One intriguing exception showed that about a third of the mortality difference between high- and low-volume hospitals for acute myocardial infarction (heart attack) could be attributed to more frequent use of proven effective medications at high-volume hospitals.

The volume of services cannot of course directly produce better outcomes. If volume is related to outcome, that association must be expressed by differences in the components of care or in the skill with which treatments are provided. For example, one study documented that high-volume surgeons were more likely to perform inappropriate carotid endarterectomies (an operation to remove or bypass a blockage in an artery narrowed by the buildup of fatty tissue) than low-volume surgeons were. Due to findings such as these, more research attention is now being paid to identifying risk variables related to the severity of the patients' presenting illness and any comorbid medical conditions that may also affect the outcomes of treatment. If high-volume hospitals treat patients who are sicker (or healthier) than their low-volume counterparts, comparisons of their outcomes are not valid without rigorous risk adjustment.

It is also evident that simply doing more operations, increasing volume, in itself is not a guarantee of superior performance. The New York State CABG study by Hannan and colleagues is a landmark example of that principle. Controlling for the effect of patient risk, they used clinical data to examine changes in surgeon volume and the relationships to mortality in New York from 1989 to 1992. They initially found that, contrary to expectations, mortality for low-volume surgeons (50 cases per year) fell 60 per cent, from 7.94 per cent to 3.20 per cent, during this period, greater than the drop observed for high-volume surgeons. Upon analysing the data further they discovered that in each year of the study the composition of the low-volume surgeon group changed markedly and could be grouped into three distinct types. One type of surgeon was moving from high to low volume as they approached retirement and reduced their workload, another was starting at low-volume and increasing as they began their careers. The third group, called persistent low-volume operators, had the poorest outcomes.

But should low volume necessarily always produce poor outcomes? Studies of heart attack data give us some idea of how better outcomes could be achieved in low-volume hospitals. For low-volume hospitals, higher mortality rates have been found among patients treated by cardiology, internal medicine and family physicians. The survival benefit in high-volume hospitals appears attributable to ensuring that patients receive the correct medication including thrombolytic agents, beta blockers and aspirin. It is obvious that key processes of care affect the volume outcome relationship. Low-volume hospitals also demonstrate greater variability because proportions based on smaller sample sizes will generate a greater chance of variability compared with larger ones. Currently we do not know how much of the observed outcome differences between high- and low-volume hospitals might be due to chance. This deficit in our knowledge is due in part to the lack of studies using longitudinal data to assess hospital or physician performance. Another consequence of the lack of longitudinal studies is the paucity of information about the shape and duration of the learning curve, either for new doctors learning standard procedures or treatments, or for experienced doctors learning new procedures. A related, rarely asked question is what level of volume is required to acquire proficiency and what level is required to retain it?

Not surprisingly, following the case of Jayant Patel, Queensland Health decided to make its medical outcome data publicly available. This could be seen as the first step toward a comprehensive undertaking to implement quality clinical auditing and consistent outcomes management, but to date this does not appear to be progressing. Rather, the data release process seems to have not taken into account the complexities of reporting this information publicly nor been informed by experience of publishing clinical indicators elsewhere. One of the main purposes of publishing clinical outcome data is so that providers can see how they do, compare themselves with their peer group, and learn and improve. Volume alone is not sufficient grounds on which to decide where procedures are carried out.

So, while much is now known about the science of improving quality of care to ensure equality between large and small providers, there is still a long way to go. And for a country such as Australia, with the challenge of preserving quality medical services in rural areas, the imperative to expand and apply outcomes management is urgent.

12

Desperately Seeking Surgeons

Australia relies heavily on overseas medical graduates. Half of its rural medical workforce is overseas trained. They work in the numerous small- and medium-sized hospitals dotted around the country's 7.7 million square kilometre expanse. With the state of Queensland covering 22.5 per cent of that land mass (second only to the sparsely populated state of Western Australia) the reliance is even stronger.

But that shouldn't mean Australia's rural population is subjected to any less a standard of individual medical practice than those who live in the city. Australia's modern healthcare system is founded on high levels of education and is seemingly well regulated. All qualified doctors, whether working in Sydney or a remote outback town, should be equally competent. Yet, with Jayant Patel, Queensland Health showed a willingness to take a doctor least likely to be fully trained, without checking his clinical performance through early supervision, and then dispatch him to a rural hospital where he continued to work with minimal or no supervision.

Throughout the investigations around Patel's behaviour it was clear that pressure is being felt within Australia's healthcare system to supply rural doctors from the pool of overseas trained applicants as there is no system to guarantee that locally trained doctors will fill those places.

And it is under pressure that cracks begin to appear.

Further exacerbating these pressures are changing trends in the make-up of the modern medical workforce. Today's state health departments such as Queensland Health are finding it harder to staff small hospitals with medical generalists. A generation ago general physicians and general surgeons were commonplace. Nowadays most physicians and surgeons sub-specialise, for instance as cardiologists or cardiac surgeons. This means that more specialists are required to be on call in any rotation period — perhaps five sub-specialists where two would have been sufficient in the past. In addition, the current generation of younger doctors contains a larger proportion of women whose time contribution to the workforce has been estimated at approximately 80 per cent of a man's. This, too, is amongst a generation where both men and women are beginning to question the wisdom of longer working hours that Australia has developed over the past 25 years at the expense of their family and social life.

There have also been changes in rural general practice, with fewer doctors willing to undertake procedural medicine such as giving anaesthetics, delivering babies and undertaking some forms of surgery. In part this is due to the huge increases in medical indemnity costs since the early 1990s driven by both court damages awards and the demise of re-insurer companies in the wake of financial downturns after the events of 9/11. Many doctors now in their 40s and 50s have left procedural practice, requiring specialist staff to support their general practice.

According to evidence heard in 2006 by the Joint Standing Committee on Migration (a bipartisan parliamentary group of the Australian Government), there were hundreds of overseas trained doctors working in Australia without anybody having assessed their skills at all. These doctors were classed as working in 'Area of Need positions' — in rural, remote and outer metropolitan hospitals — centres desperately in need of medical practitioners. These placements had increased from more than 600 in 1992. The Australian Medical Council (AMC) which administers the assessment process for overseas trained doctors seeking general registration to work in Australia also told the inquiry that specialists such as surgeons, anaesthetists and obstetricians were bypassing the formal assessment process because states and territories were using discretionary provisions to grant registration. This was despite a national agreement to involve the AMC. According to the AMC, based on Commonwealth recruitment data, in 2004 there were an estimated 790 overseas trained specialists granted temporary visas to fill Area of Need positions, but only 157 were assessed through the agreed processes.

Needless to say the council expressed its concern that it appeared medical vacancies were being hastily filled without due regard for safety and quality, clearly placing patients in danger. With the then still current media coverage about Patel, Professor John Collins, Dean of Education at the Royal Australasian College of Surgeons, set a strong tone:

> I believe that there are other potential Bundabergs out there, where people are working who have never had any assessments, and who are not under any form of appropriate supervision. We do not believe any person should be allowed to start in a position where they are going to practice without supervision. Even when assessed as capable on paper they will still need some form of supervision for a time to ensure they can perform satisfactorily in the workplace.

Ian Frank, CEO of the AMC, also pointed out that doctors who progressed through the normal medical training processes under the AMC were able, after successful completion of a Fellowship program, to be linked to continuing professional development. This was in contrast to the fate of many overseas trained doctors who often worked alone. He saw it as strange that in Australia it appeared that we were asking people to come in from overseas to go and work in often very difficult areas, culturally removed from the countries that they had come from. There was no process by which these doctors were able to integrate into the medical workforce in Australia and become effective clinicians and practitioners within the Australian healthcare system. In particular he drew attention to the experience of Canadian health authorities who also required overseas trained doctors to work in rural and remote areas. In Canada, he said:

> There are a whole lot of collateral issues around the placement of [overseas trained doctors] that go beyond simply the amount of money you pay them. Give them the support services. That is what I'm saying about the Canadians. They have identified the need to provide significant amounts of orientation and support services to back these guys up so they don't feel completely isolated.

Such forthright submissions stirred committee member Carmen Lawrence, Australia's first female Premier (1990–1993) and herself a former federal health minister, to agree that a 'proper assessment of overseas trained doctors has always been a difficult process, and it's tempting for the states to bypass it, and that's where the problems lie. What we need is a streamlined, proper, fully fledged process, which doesn't take forever, with uniform standards applied at the point of entry.' Such words indicate that least some of Australia's politicians were more than a little aware of the sometimes bewildering array of policies, guidelines, surveillance and stewardship of international medical graduates as revealed in a report submitted to the Medical Training Review Panel of the Australian Department of Health and Ageing in February 2004. Lawrence may also have been taking note of another of Ian Frank's points of contention: 'if you are going to create a national accreditation and registration system driven by bureaucracy, you'd have to say what's different to Bundaberg.'

In fact, the Australian Productivity Commission, the federal government's principal review and advisory body on microeconomic policy and regulation, had indeed recommended in 2005 for the introduction of a national accreditation board for the assessment of overseas trained doctors. Five years of wrangling the states to agree eventually resulted in the Australian Health Practitioner Regulation Agency which began operating in July 2010. The sorts of issues that must be addressed by the new agency and its supporting board include inconsistencies in terminology, a lack of national coordination in collection of data, differing entry point jurisdictions for foreign doctors, poor communication, and assessment and supervision matters. Certainly the presently inadequate resources for orientation, ongoing training and supervision of international medical graduates, and poor support for their families, will also need to be comprehensively addressed.

Some steps taken previously to streamline medical recruitment processes such as the use of contracted recruitment agencies have had their success somewhat tarnished by the revelations of the Patel case. So too might the commission's recommendations for the reduction of 'red tape' in assessment and recognition, and further flexibility in immigration arrangements to allow doctors to stay longer, be seen post-Patel as again encouraging the filling of urgent workforce needs without adequate quality control. Considering the complexities involved in the assessment process, such as diverse backgrounds and variability in knowledge and skills of overseas graduates, evaluations of competence may become reduced and formal assessments of communication skills (as distinct from linguistic proficiency) and cultural awareness may be dropped for expediency. It remains a challenging environment for the new agency and board and whether this new structure will be able to provide the efficient streamlined process that has been called for will be judged by future action.

But in the meantime things are likely to get worse rather than better, despite the growth of medical student numbers. According to Professor Lindon Wing, formerly Chair of the Committee of Deans of Australian Medical Schools, in 1988 there were 10 medical schools graduating 1200 to 1250 Australians per year. (Students from overseas do not count in relation to the Australian workforce because they had to return home after graduation.) Since then, eight new medical schools have been created and, by 2009, federally supported places had risen to approximately 2500. In addition, from 2010, all medical schools can take 25 per cent additional domestic fee-paying students which accounts for another 620. These figures do not include the fee paying students at medical schools within Australia's two private universities, Bond and Notre Dame. It also does not take into account the change in the arrangements relating to international students who can now apply to stay in Australia after graduation — currently about 50 per cent at least take internships. Overall domestic graduate numbers by 2012 are estimated to be about 3200 with at least another 200 international graduates remaining in Australia.

Yet, even with all these new graduates, Australia's ageing population means workplace shortages will progressively worsen across all states. The demographic tidal wave of baby boomers is heading towards a need for healthcare and the proportion of the working population is reducing. The reality is that we are not going to do without substantial numbers of overseas trained doctors for the next 10 years. And Australia will be competing with every other country that is also facing a medical workforce shortage.

In 2005 the *New England Journal of Medicine* published an article with the provocative title 'The metrics of the physician brain drain.' It claimed that international medical graduates constitute between 23 and 28 per cent of physicians in the United States, the United Kingdom, Canada and Australia. Medical-training positions in these developed nations, as well as opportunities for medical employment, had proved a strong draw for physicians from many nations. The origin for all those graduates was noted to be primarily India, the Philippines and Pakistan. The UK, Canada and Australia also drew a substantial number of physicians from South Africa. This physician migration (the brain drain) from source countries to recipient countries was analysed by both raw numbers and the patterns of transfer. What was clearly seen was that while a substantial transfer of physicians provided benefits in the form of services to the recipient countries and benefits in the form of remittances to the source countries, it also weakened the physician workforces of many poor nations, limiting the ability of those nations to respond to HIV infection, AIDS and other pressing medical needs. Lower-income countries contributed between 40 per cent (in Australia) and 75.2 per cent (in the UK) of the international medical graduates in recipient countries.

This reliance of the US, the UK, Canada and Australia on physicians from other nations does not preclude them from drawing on each other. Physicians from the UK constitute the largest group of international medical graduates in Canada and Australia. The US is a major recipient of physicians and loses very few. The study revealed that India has sent the most physicians to recipient countries (59,523), followed by the Philippines (18,303) and Pakistan (12,813). It was noted that limiting the negative effects of this physician drain would probably be best achieved through increased investment by recipient nations in domestic medical education. This in turn would likely decrease the amount of medical migration from poor countries and increase the medical education opportunities for citizens of recipient countries. It would also help lower-income nations to retain physicians and focus training on national needs rather than on the international physician market.

Of course, in all these statistics and predictions there remains the historical assessment by some that Australia should never have created such a reliance on overseas trained doctors in the first place. The ever frank Tony Morris, when addressing this issue himself, placed the blame on successive federal governments restricting the number of medical student places at Australian universities since the late 1980s:

> ... in 1995, [Prime Minister] Paul Keating actually reduced the total number from 1200 to 1100. He did this, not because there was any statistical reason for supposing that Australia would need fewer doctors in the future, but simply to save money for Medicare. Apparently Mr Keating and his advisers thought in simply economic terms — if you can reduce the demand for medical services, you can reduce the supply. For the next 10 years, those reductions were retained by the following [John] Howard government.

13

Something Starts to Happen

In 2006, with Patel still holed-up in his Portland home back in the US and public pressure still being applied by his victims and supporters, Queensland Premier Peter Beattie was taking a pounding in the opinion polls. Although not usually the sort of politician to worry too much about such things (he had ruled the state since 1998), this year was an election year and that could be a problem. He had already lost two safe Labor Party seats through by-elections. The Health Minister Gordon Nuttall had resigned in the wake of the Patel scandal and the media were quick to jump on any more bad news related to Queensland Health.

In August the *Courier-Mail* newspaper carried a story about Dan Naidoo, a Gold Coast health service district principal dentist who was disciplined allegedly for speaking out about a 'rogue' dentist. Naidoo was demoted and sent to a suburban dental clinic. The local MP, John-Paul Langbroek, a former dentist himself who would later go on to be state opposition leader, raised the issue in parliament, only to be told by Beattie that Naidoo had been disciplined for making inflammatory and untrue statements which would undermine public confidence in Gold Coast dental services. And according to Beattie that was that. Had Queensland Health learnt anything from the events at Bundaberg?

The last the public had heard about Patel was that the government had referred evidence to the Director of Public Prosecutions and it was likely that it would take some time to get him extradited to stand trial in Australia. Beattie's best hope was for the health scandal to die down enough before election day to restrict any swing against his party to below that needed to force a change of government.

Rob Messenger, however, was never going to make it easy for the Premier when he came visiting Messenger's Bundaberg electorate a couple of weeks out from election day. As the Premier exited his plane to walk the short distance across the airport's modest tarmac, with media crew in attendance and smiles to the ready, he was startled to hear chanting. As the media pack in front of him parted to see what was there to greet him, Beattie came face to face with the Right Honourable Member for Burnett, megaphone in hand, haranguing Beattie from behind the small chain wire fence to the side of the tarmac. Certain media commentators were later delighted to report the Premier as looking like 'a startled rabbit caught in the headlights'.

Messenger's megaphone refrain was: 'When will you bring back Patel for trial?' What Messenger didn't know at the time, but what was likely on Beattie's mind in Bundaberg, was that the Queensland Government had already rejected an offer by Patel's lawyers to voluntarily return to Australia to stand trial — a fact Beattie wanted kept secret.

It wasn't until October of 2006, after Beattie (with help from an inexperienced and bumbling opposition party) had in fact won the election convincingly, that Hedley Thomas, the same journalist who had blown the lid off the Patel story, revealed that the Queensland Director of Public Prosecutions (DPP) had agreed back in June with lawyers acting for Patel on a set of conditions for the return of Patel to face charges. Patel's lawyer in Portland, Stephen Houze, and his Brisbane counterpart Damien Scattini had worked out the details with the DPP's team led by Leanne Clare. The DPP sent a recommendation to the state Attorney-General Linda Lavarch, an elected politician, trained solicitor and a senior member of Beattie's front bench. The DPP followed up the recommendation with a supporting memo six days later, but Lavarch rejected the deal.

When the story broke, Lavarch initially said that she had not received written advice from the DPP. Later on she admitted that she had received written advice but had made the decision before it arrived. She said the decision was hers alone, and made without consulting Beattie. She explained that her reason for the rejection related to aspects of the deal that would have seen a media blackout, no further charges, no opposition to bail, and the freedom for Patel to return to the US after being charged and in between the committal hearing and the trial.

Scattini denied there was ever a claim for a media blackout and said the negotiations had been abruptly shut down. The pressure on Lavarch continued. And while Beattie angrily denounced the deal in parliament as 'sleazy', 'corrupt' and 'a rort', incensing the DPP, he also claimed that his Attorney General had failed to inform him of the existence of a strongly worded memo from the DPP recommending that the government accept the deal. Lavarch was forced to admit to misleading parliament and resigned on 13 October, citing depression. Beattie made public a letter from her psychiatrist.

The affair did little to quench the anger and frustration of those still campaigning for justice in the Patel case. It was reported that the deal would only have permitted Dr Patel to return home to the US on strict conditions including surrendering his passport and reporting to the police. In return, the privacy requested was said to only be to ensure that his flight details were not released to the press. Legal commentators expressed the view that in any case the court itself would have had the final decision about bail for Patel and he may never have been allowed out of custody anyway.

According to the media, Patel's patients were all in favour of the deal to bring him back to Australia and were quick to interpret the

Beattie government's actions as solely in its political self-interest. 'It was a political move. It was not a decision made in the best interests of patients', said Beryl Crosby, now President of the Bundaberg Patients Association. Tess Bramich, widow of the man who had been stabbed repeatedly in the chest with a catheter by Patel during bungled surgery, said in an interview with *The Australian* newspaper that all her family wanted was the closure that would come from Patel facing a criminal court. She said that the Queensland Government's continuing inability to bring back Patel from the US was causing added stress.

The spectre of political interference was never far away from the issue. Most likely, had Patel come back before the election the media would have made sure the public was reminded yet again of the failures in Queensland Health management.

When asked for her view about turning down the deal to bring back Patel, Beryl Crosby said it horrified her:

> At the end of the day I would much rather they had done that kind of deal. I still feel that Patel wants to come back; because of his arrogance, he feels he hasn't done anything wrong. I still feel that it was a political stunt. I still feel in my bones that that was politically motivated. I think that's why Linda Lavarch was so over-stressed.

On November 2006 the Brisbane Magistrate's Court finally issued a warrant for Patel's arrest on 16 charges including manslaughter, grievous bodily harm and fraud. The process of extradition could now begin. But Patel's victims would have to wait for a while yet. The process would be slow and error-prone.

In the meantime, with the clear air of three more years in power ahead of Beattie, the government was finally starting to do something about the mass of data and recommendations that had come from the previous Morris, Davies, and Forster inquiries. Queensland Health was changing. The most public commitment to change post-Patel was the promised investment of a $10 billion five-year Health Section Plan. On its website, the department published a six-month plan checklist showing progress with additional funding, pay rises for doctors, the numbers of new staff recruited, the plans for a new complaints body, clinical networks, reducing head office positions, outsourcing elective surgery to reduce waiting lists, and strengthening risk management and clinical governance.

A new Minister of Health, Stephen Robertson, and Director General of Queensland Health, Ushi Schreiber, were appointed. The executive management team was almost entirely new and included a unit called Reform and Development headed by Professor Stephen Duckett, formerly Dean of Health Sciences and Pro-Vice Chancellor for Learning and Teaching at LaTrobe University. Duckett had previously held a number of senior health positions in state and federal government including a period as Secretary for Health to the federal Keating-led government. According to Duckett, Queensland now had an opportunity that wasn't available to it pre-Patel. He saw that they could introduce safety and quality strategies that would be world-beating, by bringing onboard organisations such as the Australian Medical Association (AMA) that previously would have been reluctant. The matter of cultural change, though, was seen as a harder nut to crack. Duckett acknowledged that a range of policy domains needed to be changed and aligned to impact effectively on an organisation as large as Queensland Health. These processes of change are necessarily slow, but he believed that once the new approaches were embedded they would become the modus operandi of the organisation, reinforcing a new and different style of working together.

A crucial component to any successful change would be the newly formed Health Quality and Complaints Commission, a body independent of Queensland Health. The commission's role is to ensure that complaints and concerns about quality and safety are investigated independently. Unfortunately, the appointment of Dr John Youngman, formerly Deputy Director General of Queensland Health, as its head immediately created controversy and doubt about the new commission. Those who supported Dr Youngman pointed to his experience in quality and safety, but others pointed to his role in contributing to problems in Bundaberg by not providing a second surgeon for Dr Charles Nankivell who at the time had been working dangerously long hours and feared for the effect it could have on his patients. It was believed by many that, if the second surgeon had been appointed, there would have been no need to appoint Patel. Beryl Crosby in her position as President of the Bundaberg Patients Association was a member of the new commission. She was also critical of the appointment but continued to work with the commission.

However, Duckett was confident that, with the new complaints commission, another Patel would not be allowed to create so much havoc before being detected. In Duckett's mind the role of a whistleblower such as Toni Hoffman was now facilitated by a method of anonymous reporting that allowed multiple individual incidents to be reported. Called PRIME, the computer-based reporting system for critical incidents uses sophisticated root cause analysis on lists of sentinel events, categorising them by a Severity Assessment Code to determine the level to which they are reported in Queensland Health. The process is said to focus on what happened, why it happened, and how it can be prevented rather than who is to blame. Along with PRIME, in 2007, came the Clinician Performance Support Service based on the UK model for managing poorly performing doctors. The system provides an explicit framework for early identification of gaps in knowledge, skills, abilities or behaviours of doctors. It aims to be supportive of doctors with an emphasis on remediation at an early stage where possible and gives clinicians clarity about how to raise concerns about poorly performing colleagues. Local Directors of Medical Services remain accountable for managing poorly performing colleagues.

Changes were also made by Queensland authorities to the procedures for assessing and appointing international medical graduates. Mindful of the continuing workforce pressures, the changes focused on making recruitment even easier than before, but attempted to beef up assessment and supervision. Recruitment of some foreign doctors was in fact simplified by making use of another country's regulatory regimes. In the case of those who have already passed the UK's entry exam for overseas doctors, they are now regarded as having passed the Australian Medical Council's exam. This allows them to take out a normal Australia working visa instead of a temporary visa which prevents anyone from acquiring a mortgage or bank loan.

Specialists, however, are required by the Queensland Medical Board to undertake approximately 10 weeks of supervision and assessment, half at a major centre and half at their workplace. There is also an Australian Medical College process that requires a three-month assessment after which a specialist can then take the college exams within a year of successful completion of the assessment. Despite these initiatives there is evidence that some international medical graduates throughout 2006 and 2007 continued to be recruited *ad hoc* at a district level without a rigorous assessment, particularly in more rural areas. Such doctors would arrive at a hospital with little orientation and poor ongoing supervision of their clinical practice. The only full training program available for them is in Brisbane, sometimes thousands of miles away from their work location.

The Queensland Medical Board, stung by criticism that they held partial responsibility for Patel's rampage, also acted. They looked toward their UK colleagues and adopted a new system termed Good Medical Practice. This emphasises that the doctor's first duty is to the patients and provides specific guidance about obligations in clinical competence, observing professional obligations, good working relationships with colleagues, and probity in the conduct of business and research. Good Medical Practice makes it less likely that doctors will cover up for poorly performing colleagues, or provide inaccurate references as happened in the case of Dr Patel.

In response to criticisms throughout 2005 about the lack of consultation and communication between Queensland Health and its thousands of medical staff, Ushi Schreiber set up a Clinicians' Advisory Group which was well-received. Later it was renamed the Clinical Senate. There are mixed views about its effectiveness. New clinical networks were also set up with funds allocated to support the appointed chair. A new clinical practice improvement payment was designed to improve reporting and benchmarking by the network. However, organisational issues with the networks caused early difficulties. The use of a clinician and a non-medical professional to co-chair the networks was seen as a potential source of inefficiencies, roadblocks and over-bureaucratisation.

Local community engagement improvements were tackled via the removal of the much criticised District Health Councils and their replacement with Health Community Councils staffed to support the functions of monitoring quality, safety and effectiveness provided by the local health services. They also have a role in overseeing consumer complaints. Yet not everyone felt that the new structure was good enough to keep the politicians and bureaucrats of Queensland Health in check. The Morris Inquiry had been explicit in its description of the proper role of health boards, stating that their overriding principle is that the community should have a real sense of ownership:

> Not just symbolic ownership, but a real sense of ownership of their health system. I think the true test of whether a community does have that ownership can be found by asking, 'Is that board of local community representatives able to hire and fire the manager? Do they have direct control of the budget?' If you can't say, 'Yes' to that, I think it is going to be an ineffective body. A board that is owned by the local community is more likely to stand up to the bureaucrats and create a noise about anything untoward and let the community know about it.

14

Deadly Healthcare

Modern medical treatments save millions of lives across the globe every year, lives that were not able to be spared before the inevitable progress of science had revealed ways to formulate effective preventions and interventions.

Now science is also taking a serious look at how doctors and healthcare systems fail their patients. Over the last 15 years we have come to know much more about the extent of unintentional patient harm and how it happens. In a 2001 report on improving patient safety, Paul Barach and Fiona Moss wrote in the *British Medical Journal*: 'One guarantee that we cannot give patients is that they will not be harmed by the system that is meant to look after them.'

They went on to describe a 'silent epidemic' with startling figures. In the US, for example, they claimed that about 10 per cent of patients admitted to hospital would be harmed, with half these cases considered preventable. Of these, some 6 per cent would suffer permanent disability and 8 per cent would die. Other studies in Australia, the UK, Canada, Denmark and France have yielded similar results.

What then is the best approach to reduce medical error rates and increase patient safety?

In many cases, attempts by medical authorities over the past 10 years to implement new procedures based on reviews of errors seem stuck in what Lucian Leape calls the myth of perfection and punishment — if people try hard enough, they will not make any errors; and if we punish those who do make errors, they will make fewer of them. This flawed belief system results in people hiding their mistakes rather than learning from them. It focuses attention solely on individuals, ignoring the behavioural pressures and manipulations that occur every day within any complex social network such as a modern healthcare system.

As a number of investigations both in Australia and abroad into poor hospital patient care have shown, failure to adequately address warnings early brings about a loss of trust in administration and among clinical colleagues, and loss of trust from patients and the community. Blaming individuals or defending individuals within a sick organisational structure, rather than striving for real change, will not bring about improvements. The best way to reduce medical error rates is to target the underlying system failures that have influenced staff behaviour, rather than to just take action against individual members of a health organisation.

Professor James Reason of the University of Manchester in the UK believes that the best model of investigation and analysis of medical failures is one that improves our understanding of how systems contribute to errors. He has dubbed it the 'Swiss cheese model'. In this model, organisations naturally build into their administrative and operational systems defences, barriers and safeguards against adverse incidents to prevent errors progressing further. Ideally, each defensive layer would be intact, but in reality they are more like multiple slices of Swiss cheese with many holes, except in this case the cheese slices are somewhat 'alive', moving up and down and side to side while the actual holes in each slice also open and shut, and move their location within each slice. Accidents only occur when all the holes in the many layers line up, permitting a clear path for an accident to walk right through.

The holes in these organisational defences arise for two reasons — active failures and latent conditions. Nearly all adverse events involve a combination of both. Active failures are unsafe acts committed by people who are in direct contact with the patient or system. They may be slips, lapses, mistakes, or procedural violations. Latent conditions are the inevitable 'resident pathogens' within the system. They arise from decisions made by designers, manufacturers and top-level management. Latent conditions have two kinds of adverse effect. They can translate into error-provoking conditions such as fatigue, high workload or inadequate equipment. And they can create long-lasting holes or weaknesses in the defences. Latent conditions may lie dormant within the system for many years.

In the case of Bundaberg Hospital, latent errors can be identified as existing from early 2000, when the hospital had no credentialing and privileging committee and serious medical workforce shortages. Its controlling body, Queensland Health, ran a very centralised bureaucracy, with what was seen by many as an excessive emphasis on managing budgets, and no established procedure for dealing with poorly performing doctors. The Medical Board of Queensland itself also lacked a consistent approach to supervising the performance of overseas doctors and provided questionable checks on doctors' registration. The implementation by Queensland Health in 2006 of the independent Health Quality and Complaints Commission and PRIME reporting system can be seen as a recognition of the need to rectify these latent errors. Reducing the number of holes in the Queensland Health organisational structure would make it less likely to fail.

Applying such methods of organisational analysis as the Swiss cheese model to the realm of patient safety has highlighted the importance of transforming healthcare cultures — the shared behaviour, values and beliefs that dominate within the organisation's workforce; 'the way we do things around here'. In particular, the subset of 'safety culture' within the broader organisational culture of healthcare systems is of most concern. Safety culture relates to the beliefs and values concerning health and safety within an organisation. Early research in this area made use of assessment instruments from other industries such as aviation. Building on some of the lessons learnt in these non-medical industries and applying them to the design of safety systems in healthcare, a model that shows great promise for understanding safety culture in general practice settings is that developed by American sociologist Ron Westrum. His model allows us to understand the structure and functioning of a culture and thus to begin seeking ways to transform it.

Westrum proposed that an organisation's safety culture could be distinguished by the way in which information is handled within that organisation, and identified three different types: pathological, bureaucratic and generative. A *pathological* approach to information is power oriented and typified by: low cooperation, 'shooting the messenger', shirked responsibility, bridging discouraged, failure leading to scapegoating, and the crushing of novel ideas. A *bureaucratic* approach to information is rule oriented and typified by: modest cooperation, 'ignoring the messenger', narrow responsibilities, bridging tolerated, failure leading to justice, and novelty seen as leading to problems. A *generative* approach to information is performance oriented and typified by: high cooperation, training messengers to be effective, shared risk, bridging actively encouraged, failures leading to formal inquiry, and novel ideas leading to implementation of new systems.

Other researchers have extended this framework so that a range of safety behaviours can be identified at different levels of organisational safety culture. An example of this theoretical framework can be seen in the Manchester Patient Safety Framework now used in the UK. It uses nine dimensions of patient safety:

- Overall commitment to quality
- Priority given to patient safety

- Perceptions of the causes of patient safety incidents and their identification
- Investigating patient safety incidents
- Organisational learning following a patient safety incident
- Communication about safety issues
- Personnel management and safety issues
- Staff education and training about safety issues
- Team working around safety issues.

Through these scientific and professional advancements, the promotion and maintenance of a culture of safety has now become a prime indicator of quality in modern western healthcare systems. Such performance excellence in healthcare will be visible in any hospital or health organisation that displays a clear patient focus with visible values and high performance expectations by the organisation's senior leaders. Indeed, strong leadership in hospitals is positively associated with greater clinical involvement in quality improvement.

The challenge within Queensland Health following its tangling with Jayant Patel is to maintain an effective safety culture across all levels of patient involvement. As a first step the department has already adopted the United Kingdom NHS Leadership Qualities Framework. This leadership program, developed by the Hay Group in the UK, was almost certainly the largest ever undertaken in Australian healthcare. More than 600 top managers and clinical leaders participated in a two-and-a-half day residential workshop designed to reinforce a new approach to leadership. To follow up, a round of feedback and coaching was run to strengthen performance appraisal. A further 4500 middle managers and supervisors were also given a two-day residential workshop delivered by Queensland University of Technology. The roles of leaders were emphasised by changes to position descriptions specifically referring to accountability for patient safety and quality. A process of assessment and feedback is ongoing. A quarter of Queensland Health staff complete a culture and climate survey every six months, allowing for all staff to be surveyed within two years. The results of this survey are being fed back to District Health Services whose role is to detect where improvements in the organisational culture can be made.

The value of such organisational changes to patient safety can sometimes be underappreciated, particularly when a good scape-goating leads to a clear 'villain' being ousted from a healthcare organisation without too much scrutiny of the actual system. Yet when real change is achieved the results can be substantial. In the UK, steps toward a better culture of patient safety have not only improved healthcare standards, they have even brought about changes to medical ethics. There are now ethical obligations enforced by the UK General Medical Council that require doctors who have doubts about a colleague's professional performance to take action. A survey by the council had already determined that in the course of a professional lifetime about 50 per cent of doctors said they had concerns about a colleague and 93 per cent of them had taken some kind of action such as speaking to someone or reporting someone. In effect, the obligation for a doctor has been shifted from covering for poorly performing colleagues to putting the patient's interests first.

In practice, a doctor who is concerned about a colleague would bring it to the attention of the medical director or clinical director who has several prescribed courses of action open to them. In the first instance, after listening to all sides of the case, the medical director would want to make sure that the poor performance was not the result of illness or substance abuse, and would ask for a referral to the Occupational Health Service. If the doctor's perform-ance posed a risk to patients, he or she would be suspended on full pay or put on sick leave while the allegations were investigated. If illness was not the explanation, the medical director can choose between a disciplinary course, where there has been a violation, or a remedial course where it is a matter of technical performance. In many circumstances the solution is to move the doctor away from work that causes risks to patients into other areas where the doctor is competent; for example, teaching or administration.

Yet many of these patient safety initiatives may not have been possible in the UK without one of that country's most deadly healthcare episodes.

The tragic case of the Bristol Royal Infirmary was finally revealed by the results of a public inquiry conducted by Professor (now Sir), Ian Kennedy from University College London back in 2001. After an exhaustive three-year investigation with evidence from 577 witnesses, 900,000 pages of documentation and over 1800 medical records, many new precedents for standards of care, regulation of doctors and openness of clinical information were established. The Bristol case shows striking parallels with Patel, in particular the organisational and cultural aspects of a health bureaucracy and its clash with clinical care.

The public inquiry covered the management and care of children receiving complex cardiac surgical services at the Bristol Royal Infirmary between 1984 and 1995. The service was split between two sites, had no dedicated paediatric intensive care beds, no full-time paediatric cardiac surgeon and too few paediatric trained nurses. A statistical examination of death rates at Bristol found that they were twice the rates of other hospitals. This translated into 30 to 35 'excess deaths' at Bristol between 1991 and 1995. A detailed look at 100 operations found far more potentially serious errors in pre-operation and post-operation care than in actually doing the operation itself. About one-third of all children who underwent open-heart surgery received less than adequate care. In fact in only two types of operations did the expert assessors find that poor surgical performance was likely to have resulted in an adverse outcome.

Dr Steve Bolsin, who is now Director of Anaesthesia at Geelong Hospital in Australia, was an anaesthetist at Bristol Royal Infirmary at the time. He waged an eight-year battle to bring the scandal to light, and tearfully explained at the Kennedy Inquiry: 'in the end I just couldn't go on putting those children to sleep, with their parents present in the anaesthetic room, knowing that it was almost certain to be the last time they would see their sons or daughters alive.' After the scandal broke, Bolsin attempted to continue his medical practice but found himself ostracised by the medical establishment and was passed over for private work. He consequently left the UK to work in Australia.

Bolsin joined Bristol Royal Infirmary in 1988 from another specialised unit at Great Ormond Street Hospital in London. Immediately he noticed that operations to correct congenital heart defects in babies were taking much longer in Bristol than they should. Such delays are potentially life threatening. He began to gather data and observations and attempted to raise the matter several times via written communication with hospital executives and medical colleagues, including the president of the Association of Anaesthetists of Great Britain and Ireland. He was rebuked by the hospital executive for taking the information to 'outsiders'. Later Bolsin took minutes he had compiled from a clinical audit meeting referring to a problem with mortality rates at Bristol which he expressed as 'reaching crisis proportions', based on national mortality figures. He was told the minutes were not representative, never to produce them again and that his behaviour was 'not how we do things'. At another attempt to stir action by management at the hospital he was told 'to keep the train moving, and not to pull the communication cord'.

By 1992, across the country trainee anaesthetists and cardiac anaesthetists were all expressing concern about paediatric cardiac surgery at Bristol. Dr John Zorab, Director of Anaesthesia at another hospital in Bristol, sent a letter on Bolsin's behalf to Sir Terence English, President of the Royal College of Surgeons. The satirical magazine *Private Eye* published six articles on 'the killing fields' of Bristol, criticising the paediatric cardiac services at the hospital. Some members of a regional medical advisory group had evidence also by 1992 that Bristol was performing badly in terms of mortality, yet did not share this information with the group as a whole. The

clinicians in Bristol at least by 1990 had data on their own poor performance relative to other centres in the UK which could have
caused them at least to pause and reflect. Instead, in keeping with
the mindset of the time, they pressed on, drawing false comfort from
their figures for 1990 (which proved to be an exception). It took
another two years of complaints, lobbying and reports by Bolsin and
colleagues before was something done. In December 1994, 18-
months-old Joshua Loveday died following an operation that Bolsin
at a clinical meeting the previous day had strenuously disagreed
should be carried out. The executives at Bristol Royal Infirmary were
informed shortly thereafter that it would be inadvisable to undertake any further neonatal or infant cardiac surgery.

The Kennedy Inquiry into Bristol made 198 recommendations in
an effort to prevent a repeat of the scandal. At the outset Kennedy
himself pleaded that the National Health Service steer clear of a
culture of 'blame and shame' when implementing his findings.
Prominent among his proposals were moves to make sure that
parents (and patients) made more informed consent, and that more
public knowledge about hospital performance was available. The
inquiry adopted a systems approach to analysis in which poor performance and errors were seen as the fault of a poorly functioning
system, as much as a result of any particular individual's conduct.
He maintained that doctors who were in constant fear for their
careers might be more inclined to cover up mistakes. Bristol was a
hospital that had 'overreached itself', where clinicians had only
limited experience and were too ambitious at the time it became a
regional centre for paediatric surgery. There was a clear lack of effective clinical leadership and the management of the hospital was
flawed, with too much power in too few hands. For example, the
surgeon James Wisheart who was ultimately struck off the medical
register as a result of the inquiry was both medical director of the
hospital and chair of the hospital medical committee as well as at
various times associate clinical director of cardiac surgery and chair
of the clinical audit committee. This made open discussion and

review difficult. The body designed to respond to any concerns about doctors from staff was known as 'the three wise men'. These three executive staff were drawn from the holders of specific positions, with two of these positions held by Wisheart himself. A system of separate and virtually independent clinical directors, combined with a culture where problems were not to be brought to the chief executive for discussion and resolution, meant that there was power but no leadership. The chief executive himself saw his principal function as balancing the books. Thus, while senior managers were invited to take control and share the burden of management, there were little or no systems to monitor what they did in the exercise of that control.

Yet the culture and leadership problems promoting such a lack of healthcare safety were not restricted just to the hospitals. Kennedy also found wider problems within the NHS had contributed to the adverse patient outcomes at Bristol. There were no agreed national standards on what was good quality care for paediatric cardiac surgery, and 'while Bristol was awash with data, there was confusion in the NHS from top to bottom as to where responsibility lay for monitoring the quality of paediatric cardiac surgery'. Lacking at the very top of the UK healthcare management organisation was a systematic mechanism for monitoring clinical performance of health professionals or hospitals. Simply put, at a national level there was no single body 'keeping an eye on things'. The Supra Regional Services Advisory Group (SRSAG) thought that the health authorities or the Royal College of Surgeons was doing it; the Royal College of Surgeons thought the SRSAG or the hospital was doing it, and so it went on. The truth was that no-one was doing it.

This out of control safety management style from the very top of the healthcare organisational tree was also reflected in Wisheart's defence at the inquiry. When he sought to describe some of the factors leading to Bristol's poor outcomes, it was the NHS that featured prominently. In the late 1980s the cardiac team of just three surgeons were already working long hours day and night because of demand. Then the annual number of operations increased from 250 to 750 in just five years. Under NHS guidelines, as the number of operations increased, so did payments to the hospital. According to Wisheart, the chronic workload led the surgeons to write a memo to senior managers describing working conditions as intolerable and asking for another surgeon to be appointed. When the new surgeon arrived, management demanded that more operations be carried out, increasing the workload yet again.

In the end the Kennedy Inquiry concluded that, while adverse comments should be made about certain individuals, some of whom displayed flaws in their approach to management and a lack of leadership and insight, the lion's share of recommendations were directed at the country's national healthcare system itself. Among the recommendations made to the NHS was that they should learn from error, rather than seek someone to blame, in order to improve safety and quality. They should embrace openness and transparency as crucial to the development of trust between health professional and patient, as well as to the trust between the public and the NHS. Non executive members should play an active role in the affairs of the hospital and hospital boards must be able to lead healthcare at the local level. Continuing professional development, periodic appraisal and revalidation should be compulsory for all healthcare professionals. Senior managers should also be subject to these requirements. There was to be a new culture developed that would emphasise safety and quality, with openness and accountability and the use of collaborative teamwork; a culture of flexibility in which innovation could flourish in response to patients' needs.

In other words, less deadly healthcare.

15

Burgeoning Bureaucracy

'If Florence Nightingale were carrying her lamp through the corridors of the NHS today, she would almost certainly be searching for the people in charge.'

In 1983 the straight-talking Roy Griffiths, deputy chair and managing director of the UK supermarket chain Sainsbury's who had been appointed by Margaret Thatcher to head a government inquiry into the National Health Service, made his now famous Florence Nightingale reference. The inquiry was envisaged by the government to be a 'manpower' investigation, but soon became all about management. In Griffiths's words, 'manpower is about management, so the inquiry should be into management.'

As we have seen, the failure of management and leadership within healthcare is a common international theme across a range of investigations, inquiries and prosecutions conducted into failures of medical care over the past 25 years. And yet the size and complexity of healthcare bureaucracies continue to rise and with it the accusations and blame when things go wrong. This is strikingly so in the case of Queensland Health and Bundaberg Hospital, where sometimes quite personal and vitriolic criticism of 'faceless bureaucrats' who endangered patients was particularly strident. So where did all this extra management come from?

The UK Griffiths Inquiry is noteworthy not just for its colourful and controversial chair who released perhaps the shortest ever report from a government inquiry ever seen under a Westminster system of government — a mere 25 pages worth — but for its fundamental view that a modern government-run healthcare system needs more levels of management than available in past times. According to Griffiths, in 1983 the rapidly growing NHS had no coherent system of management at the local level. This meant that it lacked any real continuous evaluation of its performance against normal business criteria, such as levels of service, quality of product, operating within a budget, cost improvement, productivity, motivating and rewarding staff, and research and development. Precise objectives for management were rarely set and there was little measurement of health outcomes. There was little evaluation of clinical practice and even less evaluation of the effectiveness of clinical interventions.

Griffiths believed fiercely that the application of general management theory to these issues would bring about the desired changes, making the NHS a highly effective healthcare system. At the time, the NHS was operating under a type of consensus management with district management teams sharing decision responsibility amongst an administrator, medical officer, nursing officer and treasurer, all of whom had the right of veto. This approach was to be radically altered — switching the focus for decision-making onto a single individual within a hierarchy — a dramatic change.

In June the next year the government agreed to implement Griffiths's recommendations and quickly began the revamp by instituting a general manager and line managers recruited from inside and outside the NHS within each hospital. Management budgets were set and the NHS Training Authority was established to provide management training and education to doctors. The implementation was, however, never going to run smoothly. Many clinical staff baulked at what they saw as their subordination to 'supermarket-style management'. The Royal College of Nursing mounted a campaign to resist general managers, seeing in the change a significant downgrading of their influence in patient care decision-making.

The new general managers were to be operationally and professionally accountable to their counterparts at district level. The intention was to call for active strategic direction and real responsibility through a clear line of management and devolved budgets. A crucial element in the introduction of general management was the recognition of the need to find a way of involving doctors, particularly senior doctors, in the day-to-day management of the NHS. Several models had already been tried previously, yet this time the NHS also had the benefit of Professor (later Sir) Cyril Chantler of the United Medical Schools of Guy's and St Thomas' Hospitals in London who promoted the use of a 'clinical directorate' model developed earlier in the US at Johns Hopkins Hospital in Baltimore in 1972.

The clinical directorates model suggested that clinical services should be organised in a series of directorates. Each directorate would have a clinical director or lead consultant, usually chosen by the other doctors within the directorate, to act for them with hospital management. The clinical director was expected to assume responsibility for providing leadership to the directorate and to represent the views of the clinical specialty. They would also initiate change, agree on work plans and resource allocation with the unit general manager, and act as the budget holder for the directorate. The relationship between the clinical director and colleagues was not, however, to be viewed as one of line management. Instead, the clinical director was expected to achieve results through the negotiation and persuasion of their colleagues. All NHS staff were also expected to focus on producing satisfied customers or consumers, a view in direct contrast to that previously held — that patient outcomes were solely the preserve of healthcare professionals.

While today no-one in the UK disputes that the 1980s shift toward more professional management benefited the NHS, there remains resentment over the appointments and rapid rises in pay and influence granted to the new bureaucracy, and the way the process was seen to alienate medical staff from managers. It can be argued that a fundamental difficulty with implementing the Griffiths Inquiry report rests on the simple fact that a hospital is not a commercial business. No major incentives were available to persuade those working in the NHS to change their ways of working. Nor would any competitive pressure from a public marketplace bring economic sanctions for poor performance. If a commercial endeavour fails to perform adequately it is taken over or goes out of business. A hospital cannot be shut down, and, no matter what, it has to continue to offer a service.

Back in Australia, the effect of the NHS overhaul was to encourage most state and territory health services in Australia to also follow suit and begin applying various models of general management, adding new layers of health bureaucracy. Queensland Health took to the idea of increased management with particular enthusiasm, spreading its regional district managers across the expansive state. Getting accurate figures on the total workforce of Queensland Health has in the past been somewhat difficult given the department's reputation for secrecy, but since a highly publicised payroll bungle in 2010 it is now acknowledged that the department employs around 77,000 people. The number of doctors in 2007 was stated to be 5601.

According to Tony Morris it was precisely the structure of Queensland Health's new layers of bureaucracy that were to blame in a large part for the extent of the havoc wrought by Patel, rather than those individuals who worked within them. He believes that District Managers, Directors of Medical Services and others are not expected to think for themselves, and in fact are not even allowed to. Unlike private-sector employers — who look for managerial staff who are resourceful, who have judgment and discretion, presence of mind, show initiative, and are innovative, progressive and proactive

— Morris believed these qualities often appeared to disqualify a person from appointment or promotion within the Queensland Health bureaucracy. Thus, in his mind, the executives in Bundaberg in 2003 did exactly what was expected of them — no more, no less — and the real blame lies with the architects of the system which set them up to fail. Morris was, however, still scathing in his assessment of senior bureaucratic talent in the department:

> Even the calibre of the bureaucrats inhabiting the executive offices of Bundaberg Base Hospital — itself a very significant contributing factor to the Patel phenomenon — was merely symptomatic of a far more fundamental malaise within Queensland Health. People of that character, occupying such positions, are not employed by chance. From my observation, most of these individuals would not even make the short list for the manager of a McDonald's hamburger restaurant.

Not surprisingly, then, Morris remained unconvinced that general management theory is the way forward for modern healthcare systems. He enlisted examples from other branches of government and from private enterprise to support his arguments illustrating how these other enterprises are under the control of people who are experts in the organisation's core functions, 'not experts at bean counting and paper shuffling'. In police stations, administrative staff report to the senior police officer, not the other way around. In schools and universities the top executive positions are held by vice chancellors whose expertise is education, not business management. Law courts are headed by a senior judge or magistrate. The Chief Justice or Chief Magistrate is not told how to run his court by an administrative functionary. The Undersecretary of the Department of Foreign Affairs is a senior diplomat, not a bureaucrat. According to Morris:

> Only in the healthcare sector have experts — the medical practitioners and other healthcare professionals — allowed their control of their own working environment to be taken over by people who have no relevant expertise or qualifications. Doctors who spend 70 hours a week looking after patients are no match for bureaucrats who spent 40 hours a week looking after themselves.

Despite this somewhat pessimistic view, or indeed perhaps because of such observations, a 2006 Queensland Health management restructure was introduced to try and shift care accountability from District Manager up through the Area Manager to the Director General. The Patient Safety and Quality Board was instituted to be made up of the Director General, the three area managers, and six members appointed after consultation with external organisations, including consumers. In this regard Queensland Health continues to follow the NHS model but without such a clear link between clinicians and managers acting through the role of the directors of medical services. In essence, managers in Queensland were being given responsibility but without the technical clinical knowledge to be able to fully understand the issues. The Patient Safety Centre operates through District Patient Safety Officers with post descriptions and service-level agreements between the Patient Safety Centre and the Districts. This ensures that the funding for the post does not get used for other purposes. The Patient Safety Officers are, however, a valuable resource to support clinicians and managers in improving patient safety, and serve three main functions: education and training for staff in patient safety; district compliance with clinical incident management policies, particularly for serious adverse events; and evaluation and auditing of safety improvement activities.

Queensland Health has also created four new posts for Clinical CEOs. Bill Beresford, the man originally given the role to 'fix' Bundaberg post-Patel, took up one such position, that of District Manager for central Queensland district. His first task was to implement a district operational plan for clinical risk management. Believing that long hours on duty contribute to medical mishaps, Dr Beresford substantially increased the staff at Rockhampton by attracting full-time staff while also chartering aircraft to fly specialists out to do sessions at smaller rural centres. He also supported the isolated doctors in more remote areas by using fly-in specialists to work with the local doctor for selected medical services. Not only does this ensure a safer service but it keeps the rural doctor's skills up-to-date and under supervision. Beresford is also looking at other clinical governance issues to support the lone rural doctor, such as re-credentialing them based on their attendance at Maintenance of Professional Standards programs, numbers of procedures undertaken and their outcomes, and other forms of appraisal.

In contrast to Morris's pessimism, these sophisticated initiatives from a new level of management which should lead to better healthcare outcomes for Queensland Health. But their success will surely be due more to the fact that an experienced clinician has been given a senior management role — not that management theory itself has brought better outcomes to the practice of modern healthcare.

16

A Matter of Judgment

The view from Jayant Patel's cell in the Los Angeles Metropolitan Detention Centre on 17 July 2008 was said to be less than salubrious, overlooking the city's down market downtown area bordered by the congested Hollywood Freeway. He had been moved suddenly from his Portland jail cell by US Marshalls under a 'sealed' order of US District Court Judge Dennis Hubel just before dawn to begin the journey back to Australia and the Australian judicial system. It was now four months since the FBI had appeared at his home in the affluent suburb of Raleigh Hills early in the morning and taken him into custody. It was a staggering 19 months since the Brisbane Magistrate's Court had issued his arrest warrant. It was to be nearly another year and a half before he was found guilty.

The US Marshalls' move to take Patel to Los Angeles had the same air of controversy that had dogged the DPP's efforts for extradition since November 2006. The event caught many by surprise. Details were sketchy because of the court ruling for secrecy and the Australian media scrambled to find out when exactly Patel would be put on a plane for Brisbane. Patel's supporters began claiming that the then US Secretary of State Condoleezza Rice was being pressured by the Australian Government to sign the final extradition papers within a shortened deadline. The US Marshalls and Los Angeles detention authorities were tight lipped.

In truth, the legal and procedural moves were the surprisingly well-coordinated end to a lengthy error-prone process of extradition. A reported six drafts were sent by the DPP over 16 months after the Australian issue of his warrant for arrest before the US Department of Justice lodged the final application allowing his arrest in Portland.

Patel's lawyers immediately opposed the extradition, winning the right to examine detailed medical records of the patients he was accused of harming, and delaying extradition processes with allegations of 'bungled' paperwork by Queensland police. It seemed the case would drag on for years, before suddenly in June 2008 they dropped their objection, stating that Patel was willing and desirous of returning to Australia to contest the allegations against him. They asked that he be allowed to return home to his wife Kishoree until the extradition proceedings were finalised and be monitored by a global positioning system by authorities. The court refused and he remained in jail until the US Marshalls roused him from his bed in July.

Patel flew into Brisbane from Los Angeles on a Qantas flight accompanied by two Australian detectives, arriving on Monday 21 July 2008 and was released on bail of $20,000 by the Brisbane magistrate. He was ordered not to approach any witnesses in the case against him, not to leave the secret address approved by the magistrate or leave Queensland without written permission. He was charged with 14 offences including three counts of manslaughter, one of causing grievous bodily harm, one of committing negligent acts causing harm, and fraud.

After a committal hearing of a little over two months, Jayant Patel finally came to trial in the Supreme Court in Brisbane on 23 March 2010. By then, after lengthy legal argument, the fraud charges had been held over for a separate trial and he faced three charges of manslaughter and one of grievous bodily harm. All the victims were patients on whom Patel had operated. James Edward Phillips, a 46-year-old man in end-stage renal failure, died after Patel performed surgery on him to remove part of his oesophagus for cancer. Gerardus Kemps, 77, also died after Patel conducted an oesophagectomy but failed to control internal bleeding. Patel removed part of the bowel of Mervyn Morris, 75, who died of post-operative complications. Ian Vowles, then 62, had his colon removed by Patel, leaving him with a colostomy bag. Patel pleaded not guilty to all four charges.

From the start the trial set legal precedent. Judge John Byrne allowed the trial to be televised live into a Bundaberg courthouse. This was the first time in Australian legal history that a major trial was to be televised. Tony Morris was an enthusiastic supporter of the move, seeing it as providing those people most affected by the case with the ability to view proceedings and gain insight into what happens in a courtroom. He remains reserved, however, as do most Australian criminal law practitioners, about any moves to expand public access to ongoing criminal trials. The American style of justice with its media frenzies of lawyers standing on courthouse steps explaining tactics and strategies is not the Australian way.

But, even as Prosecutor Ross Martin SC opened the case for the Crown, controversy dogged the proceedings. One of three reserve jurors was allowed to leave on the first day after expressing concerns over whether he could remain impartial. Another juror was permitted to talk with the judge about his own concerns about impartiality but was allowed to remain. Two days later, a second juror was discharged after a note was sent to the judge. (The details of the note, seen by both the prosecution and defense, were not revealed, and the reasons may have been unrelated to the case.) Five days following this it was revealed that one of the serving jurors was an employee of Queensland Health and they were duly discharged. With only one juror now held in reserve, there were concerns two weeks later when another juror fell ill, and proceedings were adjourned for four days.

The prosecution's case for criminal negligence was seen from the outset as a difficult one to prove. It is not a popular option for Australian prosecutors. Australia's last conviction for medical manslaughter was in 1843 when Dr William Valentine of Campbelltown, New South Wales, gave a bottle to young Robert Aiken to deliver to a sick patient of his, Theophilus Swifte. A short while after receiving the bottle, Swifte commented to his teaching colleagues at breakfast that he had awoken not feeling at all well but after taking a dose of medicine was now feeling very strange indeed. He commented that the medicine had tasted bitter and unlike anything he had had previously. He felt as if he had been drinking brandy and was very light headed. He soon collapsed. Dr Valentine was called for and for the next seven and half hours he worked to try and save Swifte. When summoned, Valentine had brought with him a stomach pump and stated to others at the scene that when he heard Swifte had fainted he realised that he had made a mistake and given Robert Aitken the wrong bottle from his surgery table. Instead of a black draught (a common 19th century purgative) he had inadvertently picked up a similar sized bottle of laudanum (an opium preparation). The court case featured numerous witnesses testifying to Valentine's kind nature, his professional manner, and appropriateness of his methods to try and save Swifte's life. The court also heard of the labelling details of the two medicines and their placement in Valentine's surgery. Valentine was found guilty but strongly recommended to the mercy of the court. He was sentenced to a fine of 25 pounds.

Patel, however, was not to have the benefit of a string of witnesses testifying to his kind nature. Rather, this was a case about his medical capability. The prosecution sought to show that Patel had carried out operations without reasonable skill and care and was thus liable under Section 288 of the Queensland Criminal Code. The defence, led by Michael Byrne QC, brought in a range of expert medical witnesses to testify that Patel's surgery was not the cause of the patient's deaths, but rather complications after surgery, and noted that all patients had given consent for the surgery.

As the trial progressed, it became obvious that the prosecution were struggling to show that Patel had acted carelessly. He might not have been a great surgeon, but there was little evidence that his surgical technique was all bad. They attempted to bolster their argument by reminding the jury of the failure by Wavelength and the Queensland Medical Board to identify Patel's operating restrictions in Oregon, the doubtful appointment of Patel as Director of Surgery in Bundaberg, and Queensland Health's policy of not transferring patients to Brisbane. Evidence on hospital underfunding, how Patel's prodigious operating schedule brought in considerable funds to the hospital, and medical director Darren Keating's alleged failure to act on the concerns of Toni Hoffman and Peter Miach was also presented.

The jury heard about Patel's 'toxic ego' as the prosecution painted a picture of Patel as a man driven to prove others wrong: 'It is easy to see, when you know all the evidence, how ambition, ego and a lack of insight will lead a man stung by the order of Oregon to prove himself, redeem himself in his own eyes.'

Yet under Section 288, all this prosecution testimony was irrelevant. The prosecution's case was falling apart as the defence argued that under law the matter to consider was confined to incompetence in doing surgery to which the patient consented. The case was not about the witnesses or Patel's personality but about the roles of doctors in relation to the criminal code. When the prosecution tried to change its case midstream to another section of the Criminal Code the judge rejected it. Forced to continue, Martin then set about extending the interpretation of what is a relatively old provision of the Queensland Criminal Code into realms never before chartered. He now argued that while Patel may have been legally permitted to operate on patients who had given consent and done so adequately, it was his decision to operate that was negligent, rather than the act of surgery itself. Despite a vigorous attack on this position by the defence, Justice Bryne ruled that such an interpretation was preferable:

> The accused is not absolved from criminal responsibility for the adverse outcomes to his patients merely because he had their consent for the procedures and, if it be the fact, performed them with reasonable skill and care.

The judge said he found it remarkable that after 110 years of law the operation of Section 288 had not been more closely examined.

The trial had been turned on its head. And most of this legal argument had occurred out of the eyes and ears of the jury, in chamber discussions. The defence now realised the harm to their own case that the prosecution's evidence about Patel's behaviour outside of the operating theatre had caused, and applied to the judge to discharge the jury on the grounds of inadmissible and prejudicial evidence. Justice Byrne denied the request and said that it could be resolved by proper and adequate directions to the jury.

Patel was not called to give evidence in his defence.

In his summing up to the jury, Justice Byrne said that the trial was not about 'botched surgery' but rather about Patel's judgment in deciding to perform the operations and whether it showed 'such serious disregard of the patients' welfare that he should be punished as a criminal'. 'Or in other words that his decision to operate was so thoroughly reprehensible, involving such great moral guilt, that it should be treated as a crime deserving punishment.'

After six and a half days of deliberation, on 29 June 2010 the jury returned its verdict of guilty on all three counts of manslaughter and one count of grievous bodily harm. Patel was sentenced the day after to seven years on each of the manslaughter counts and three years on account of grievous bodily harm, to be served concurrently. The judge took into account that Patel would have special difficulties in prison because of his notoriety, had served some time already, and that he had no criminal history.

The guilty verdict immediately raised concerns amongst both the legal and medical fraternity. To some commentators the decision was surely destined to be overturned by a higher court. For others it represented a ground-breaking precedent. Doctors worried that they might now be found criminally liable for adverse outcomes stemming from operations and the decisions they made, thus driving up medical insurance costs.

Yet Justice Byrne himself made clear in his Court that Patel knew very well that he was deciding to perform operations in Bundaberg that he had been restricted from practising in the United States by an order of the local Board of Medical Examiners. It was reasonable to accept also that the reasons for these restrictions related to deficiencies in his knowledge. Patel was also required by the US medical authorities to get a second opinion before undertaking complicated surgery, oesophageal surgery, and surgery on high-risk patients with severe comorbidities — requirements not revealed to his Australian patients and the Bundaberg hospital. These specific elements of the case appeared likely to restrict the use of the Patel decision in setting any legal precedent. Judge Byrne himself was quoted as saying that 'no one would be a surgeon if the criminal law did not afford protection to a surgeon when things went wrong.'

Patel's lawyers however not surprisingly lodged an appeal a couple of weeks later claiming that a number of Justice Byrne's judicial rulings during the trial were erroneous and had thus resulted in a miscarriage of justice. Central to their claim was argument over the mid-trial change in the Crown's case and the resultant effect on evidence previously presented. But no sooner had Patel's legal team begun preparing for a scheduled November appeal hearing when yet another roadblock surfaced. Patel was running out of money. He had benefitted from respected and high calibre legal representation that had worked hard for their client. But such work didn't come cheap. The Court of Appeal was asked to delay the hearing while 'funding issues' were worked out.

Meanwhile, the Queensland Government was also busy with legal fees. Only three days after the announcement of Patel's appeal, Attorney-General Cameron Dick announced they were lodging their own appeal against Patel's seven-year prison sentence, maintaining that it was inadequate and failed to reflect the gravity of the offences. It was clear the government wanted to keep Patel behind bars.

By October 15, when mention of Patel's appeal was next before the Court, both his Solicitor, Arun Raniga, and his then Barrister, Michael Woodford, informed Court of Appeal President Margaret McMurdo that Patel had been unable to reach an agreement with them about payment and that Patel had formally applied for funding to Legal Aid Queensland (LAQ), an independent government funded body which provides legal assistance to the economically and socially disadvantaged. The decision on funding was still underway and had necessitated consideration of Kishoree Patel's financial affairs. Justice McMurdo reiterated her earlier concern that the Court hear Patel's appeal earlier rather than later but was forced to again put off consideration of the case for another mention the next month.

It wasn't looking good for Patel. In fact, when Justice McMurdo faced Patel's legal counsel on November 12, she was informed that the LAQ had just 24 hours earlier refused Patel's aid request. Arun Raniga sought leave to withdraw as a result but announced that the appeal would still go ahead under a new legal team still being assembled. Patel was then represented by Andrew Boe, a Brisbane-based lawyer who shot to national prominence in the mid nineteen nineties when as a young solicitor in New South Wales he took on the task of defending Ivan Milat, later jailed for life as Australia's notorious backpaker serial killer. Mr Boe no longer sported the full head of long flowing black hair that ran past his shoulders all those years ago and was now standing as a Barrister with a reputation as a fearless and passionate advocate for appellate review. Patel's appeal was tentatively set down for early February.

Yet, still the case would twist.

A scant 12 days later, it was not Andrew Boe standing beside Jayant Patel at the 10 minute Court of Appeal hearing on November 24, but, Ken Fleming QC, who now told Justice McMurdo that he was anxious for the matter to be heard. Mr Fleming had worked as a public servant and farmer before studying law and eventually 'taking silk' as a Queen's Counsel in 1988. He is known as one of the state's most experienced lawyers with an intricate knowledge of the law, having served with the United Nations as a prosecutor for crimes conducted during upheavals in Rwanda and Sierra Leone that had cost many innocent lives. His services would normally not come cheap. In Patel's case they came free — pro bono publico.

On March 3, 2011, Mr Fleming, backed by a reported 5 barristers, argued that Patel's trial had been 'allowed to run amok' when prosecutors had changed tack mid-trial. Patel himself sat stony faced, jotting down notes as argument continued. Mr Fleming presented to the court that after 39 days of the original trial it became clear Patel would not be convicted of causing the deaths as a result of the actual operations because the prosecutors had failed to show that the operations themselves caused the deaths or injury. It was then that they moved the goal posts with the decision to change which part of the law their case was relying on. By that time, according to Mr Flemming, the jury had heard evidence about the actual surgery and Patel's past conflicts with authorities in the US, that was so prejudicial no adequate directions by the judge could remedy it. This argument was opposed by Ross Martin SC, still presenting the crown's case, who instead said that the mid-trial change had in fact made it more difficult for the prosecution to successfully pursue its case.

Both parties argued strongly before the Court's three senior judges during the three day hearing, giving little ground. It took another 6 weeks of consideration before a 60-page judgment was finally released on April 21, 2011. In a unanimous decision the Court dismissed Patel's appeal, finding that there had been no miscarriage of justice in the verdicts and no 'material irregularity or unfairness' in the conduct of the trial. The judges noted again the fact that Patel had been under notice not to perform complicated surgery by a medical board in Oregon and as such his limitations as a surgeon and his understanding of those limitations were relevant to any interpretation of his conduct as involving 'grave moral guilt'. The court was also unimpressed by the Government's attempts to extend Patel's time in jail, declaring that the sentence 'properly balances the exacerbating and mitigating feature of this unique case and was not manifestly excessive.'

Reaction to Patel's jailing was mixed. Gerry Kemps' widow Judy said her only concern was the guilty verdict and not the amount of time that he would spend in jail. Beryl Crosby was relieved that the six-year fight was over. For Beryl, too, it was a guilty verdict that mattered, not the sentence. Toni Hoffman was 'over the moon' and relieved. She also thought the sentence wasn't important. Queensland Health did not give Toni special leave to attend the trial or any of the other related activities, including the committal proceedings and the Royal Commission. She had used all of her leave entitlements over the previous five years in following and assisting in investigations.

Rob Messenger thought the sentence was totally inadequate, as did a number of the victim's families.

17

The Aftermath

In January 2011 as we write, Bundaberg is now managed from a district headquarters 263 kilometres away at Nambour and is part of the Sunshine Coast district. There are no historical connections culturally or administratively between the medical administrations of Bundaberg and Nambour. The local Cluster Manager (a new term) is shared with Hervey Bay 80 kilometres away. The hospital has no Director of Medical Services of its own, instead sharing the position with the director at Hervey Bay. Only recently has the post occupied by Patel, Director of Surgery, been filled. Queensland Health was apparently unwilling to compete in the international market to fill this sensitive position. The Davies Inquiry report and its recommendations for improving health outcomes has been removed from the Queensland Health website.

When Ushi Schreiber left Queensland Health in 2007 she had completed a reorganisation of state health services which saw 37 health districts merge into 20, and the Bundaberg Base Hospital becoming part of the Wide Bay District and dropping the 'Base' from its name. Her role was left unfilled for a while before Mick

Reid, a career bureaucrat, was recruited from minister Nicola Roxon's office at the Federal Department of Health and Ageing in Canberra. He has initiated another reorganisation in which the number of health districts has been further reduced to 15, although the reasons behind this reorganisation in contrast to that of Schreiber's are unclear.

This apparent penchant of Queensland Health for restructures is a worrying aspect of the government's ultimate response to the lessons presented by the Patel case. Change is not always for the better. Regular changes can be downright dangerous.

The UK's NHS Confederation, which has seen 16 reorganisations in 30 years, recently reported on the outcomes of all that reorganisation. Their findings were not encouraging. Similar to the commercial sector, where only 25 to 30 per cent of mergers succeed, they found the complexity and risk involved with health services more often than not brought about dysfunctional effects. Downsides of reorganisation included a loss of focus on patient services, increased risks to patient safety, increased inertia in the organisation, dislocation of key external relationships and difficulties in transferring good practice within the merged organisation. Savings were seldom achieved, and promised benefits rarely realised. The value of mergers in particular was challenged by the NHS review with the finding of only sparse evidence of scale advantages:

> … the relatively poor performance of some of the very large organisations created in this way suggests that these are over stated. It seems likely that the marginal costs of additional complexity may increase more rapidly than any advantages from increased scope and scale.

Why then do reorganisations occur? They can certainly be popular with individual managers and senior bureaucrats who can see a chance of more highly paid positions. Even 'losers' in a merger, if senior enough, can benefit from substantial retirement and severance salary packages. For government policy makers, 'structural change' is one the few devices that allows them to intervene in the specialised world of clinical decision-making. It also allows difficult decisions to be avoided while providing a defence against allegations of inaction. Reorganisation can bring about the removal of troublesome senior staff and is a highly publicly visible activity for governments and organisations, displaying the clear message that something is being done. This is particularly the case where a merger or acquisition is used to deal with organisational failure. Yet if this reorganisation fails, or is seen to be not achieving results quick enough, it usually sparks another round of structural changes. Researchers have argued that this approach to health restructuring is based on a formal, hierarchical and mechanistic view of how organisations work — that, through centralised planning, command and control, effective change will automatically ensue. It underestimates the importance of culture, norms, values and relationships.

Speaking to people who have been in and around Queensland Health since 2005, one can't escape the conclusion that things only got better temporarily and that ongoing organisational restructures and mergers are taking their toll. Many feel everything has reverted to the old style of top-down management and are fearful to speak out. Morale is said to be going down. Martin Strahan had had enough of Queensland Health by mid 2009 and resigned as Director of Medicine at Bundaberg Hospital. In his opinion the new changes to the state health system such as clinical networks appeared to be Brisbane-centric activities with little relevance to Bundaberg.

Rob Messenger has noted that an emergency department nurse at Bundaberg Hospital, Christine Cameron, reported incidents in the emergency department using the new PRIME system only to find those reports were ignored. She got little satisfaction from Queensland Health, blew the whistle, and now is on long-term stress leave. She appears to have been vindicated by the belated building of a $6 million improved emergency department. PRIME may not be the protection against the Patels of this world that Stephen Duckett had hoped for, nor according to Rob Messenger is the Health Quality and Complaints Commission which frequently sends complaints back to Queensland Health rather than completing an independent inquiry.

And how is the new system handling complaints and difficulties? In late November 2009 Bundaberg Hospital faced another scandal when it was revealed that as many as 235 people might have been exposed to dangerous pathogens and blood diseases such as HIV after a dental health clinic sterilising machine was accidently left turned off for a week and unsterilised instruments removed from it and used. The Deputy Premier, Paul Lucas, arrived in Bundaberg declaring that 'heads will roll'. It took Beryl Crosby to counsel him that such an attitude was precisely what they were now trying to avoid. As she told him: 'If you talk like that, people won't own up, and we want get to the bottom of things so that we can avoid the same mistakes in the future.' The person who operated the steriliser was fired just the same — a convenient scapegoat perhaps.

After the trial verdict on Patel, Queensland Health was quick to claim through the media that lessons had been learnt, the system improved and that these problems were in the past. Peter Beattie, now retired, wrote an article in *The Australian* newspaper placing the blame for Bundaberg on the lack of oversight by the Queensland Medical Board and an insufficient supply of doctors. Michael Wooldridge, Commonwealth Health Minister from 1996 to 2001, wrote a stinging rebuttal under the headline of 'Beattie must not shift blame to others for the Bundaberg disaster'. Wooldridge wrote that 'to those of us who operated on a national level, there was not the slightest surprise that when the disaster occurred, it happened in Queensland.' In his time as health minister he said it was always clear that the state with the most centralised, bureaucratic and 'Stalinist' health service was Queensland. He claimed Queensland Health operated in a climate of abject terror and that under Beattie, first as health minister then as premier, you had to 'keep your numbers up': 'As an administrator, you were judged on it and you received a bonus if you achieved it. Thus, a doctor, hospital or health bureaucrat that performed unnecessary or questionable surgery was given a bonus.'

While Wooldridge admitted that Patel was indeed a tragedy for Bundaberg, he believed he had 'walked into an environment tailor-made for the disaster to occur'.

The aftermath of the Jayant Patel case leaves a substantial personal, medical, legal and economic impact. Nearly 400 former patients of Jayant Patel sought compensation with the Queensland Government, and almost three-quarters have settled their claims. Beryl Crosby, President of the Bundaberg Patients' Association, feels that the compensation process has gone well in all but a few instances. The government has paid for the claimants' legal expenses and the settlements are, in her view, more generous than might have been obtained through the courts. Rob Messenger disagrees. He says that patients and relatives were made to sign confidentiality agreements before they could access the mediation process. He believes that spouses received $8000 compensation — about the same as the fee earned by the lawyer. The Queensland Government has consistently refused to disclose how much money has gone into compensation. Some victims are considering a class action against Queensland Health.

Toni Hoffman, who has met the Queen and the Prime Minister and been awarded the Local Hero award for her courageous whistle-blowing work, has now returned as Charge Nurse of the ICU at Bundaberg Hospital. Rob Messenger retained his seat during the election and introduced a Private Member's Bill to protect whistle-blowers, which was defeated. A later government bill on whistle-blowing was passed and protective legislation now exists. Peter Leck became a medical student and Darren Keating returned to WA to practise as a GP. The Queensland authorities decided not to pursue criminal charges against him. Dr Bill Beresford retired to WA from his Rockhampton Queensland Health post in 2008. In March 2009, Stephen Duckett left Australia to become the President and Chief Executive Officer of Alberta Health Services, Canada, until being controversially sacked for a highly publicised on-camera media exchange where he expressed the desire to keep eating his cookie rather than answer a reporter's questions.

Thus, while there has been closure for many of Patel's victims and others such as Toni Hoffman, doubts remain about how much the management and structure of Queensland Health has changed for the good. Both Rob Messenger and Martin Strahan agree that one good thing is that health expenditure in Queensland has almost doubled since the time of Patel. New facilities have been built and there are twice as many doctors. The main beneficial outcome for Beryl Crosby has been the establishment of Health Consumers Queensland along with the Patient Safety Centre. This initiative she feels has succeeded in bringing about mandatory reporting of poorly performing doctors and open disclosure when something has gone wrong, with a subsequent increase in critical incident reporting.

But there are many who believe that the lessons to be learnt from the Patel case by Queensland Health, and indeed by healthcare systems elsewhere in Australia and overseas, are not being given the attention they deserve. Real change is often difficult to achieve and the convenience of 'kicking heads', scapegoating, and the use of public relations expertise to smooth over cracks, are modern management techniques employed all too quickly. Yet we ignore the lessons at our peril.

The story of Jayant Patel, Bundaberg Hospital and Queensland Health is relevant for all who are a part of a modern, complex healthcare network, from hospital administrators to doctors, nurses, ancillary staff and the patients themselves. The case of the infamous 'Dr Death' could be happening again right now in your own modern overburdened healthcare system.

Bibliography

Chapter 1

Thomas H. Sick to death. Sydney: Allen and Unwin, 2007.

The Oregonian. PDF documents including results of Oregon Medical Board reports, letters of praise from colleagues at Kaiser, job references, and letters of recommendation from Dr J Raymond Hinshaw of University of Rochester. Unfortunately some of the links are now dead. Accessed 28 January 2007 at http://www.oregonlive.com/oregonian/malpractice/?/oregonian/malpractice/stories/storiesindex

Hansard. 16 March 2006. http://www.aph.gov.au/hansard. The Standing Committee on Health and Ageing of the House of Representatives placed the Morris Enquiry report on record so that it was not lost from history.

Final Report of the Queensland Public Hospitals Commission of Inquiry (The Davies Report). Accessed October 2010 at www.qphci.qld.gov.au

Queensland Health Systems Review. Final Report (the Forster Report) available at www.health.qld.gov.au

Mullan F. The metrics of the physician brain drain. NEJM 2005;353:1810–1818.

Loy CS, Warton RB, Dunbar JA. Workforce trends in specialist and GP obstetric practice in Victoria. Med J Austral 2007;186:26-30.

Emslie S, Knox K, Pickstone M, eds. Improving patient safety: insights from American, Australian and British healthcare. London: ECRI &DH, 2002.

Walshe K, Shortell SM. When things go wrong: How healthcare organisations deal with major fauliures. Health Affairs 2004;23:103–111.

Berwick DM. Not again! BMJ 2001;322:247–248.

An Organization with a Memory: Department of Health, London. Accessed July 2006 at www.dh.gov.uk/publicationsandstatistics/publications/publicationspolicyandguidance.

Wolff, A, Taylor, S. Enhancing patient care: a practical guide to improving quality and safety in hospitals. Strawberry Hills, NSW: MJA Books, 2009.

Chapter 2

Child A, Glover P. Report on obstetric and gynaecological services at KEM and the Metropolitan Health Service Board, WA 2004.

Dunbar JA, Reddy P. Beresford B, Ramsey WP, Lord RSA. In the wake of hospital inquiries: impact on staff and safety. Med J Aust 2007;186:80–83.

Hansard. 16 March 2006. http://www.aph.gov.au/hansard. The Standing Committee on Health and Ageing of the House of Representatives placed the Morris Enquiry report on record so that it was not lost from history.

Final Report of the Queensland Public Hospitals Commission of Inquiry. (The Davies Report). Available at www.qphci.qld.gov.au. Accessed October 2010.

The Oregonian. PDF documents including results of Oregon Medical Board reports, letters of praise from colleagues at Kaiser, job references, and letters of recommendation from Dr. J. Raymond Hinshaw of University of Rochester. Accessed on 28th of January 2007 http://www.oregonlive.com/oregonian/malpractice/?/oregonian/malpractice/stories/storiesindex.html

Chapter 3

Hansard. 16 March 2006. http://www.aph.gov.au/hansard. The Standing Committee on Health and Ageing of the House of Representatives placed the Morris Enquiry report on record so that it was not lost from history.

Final Report of the Queensland Public Hospitals Commission of Inquiry (The Davies Report). Accessed October 2010 at www.qphci.qld.gov.au

Queensland Health Systems Review. Final Report (the Forster Report). Accessed October 2010 at www.health.qld.gov.au

Thomas H. Sick to death. Sydney: Allen and Unwin, 2007.

Chapter 4

Thomas H. Sick to death. Sydney: Allen and Unwin, 2007.

The Oregonian. PDF documents including results of New York and Oregon medical board reports, letters of praise from colleagues at Kaiser, job references, and letters of recommendation from Dr J Raymond Hinshaw of University of Rochester. Accessed October 2010 at http://www.oregonlive.com/oregonian/malpractice/?/oregonian/malpractice/stories/storiesindex

Chapter 5

Hansard. 16 March 2006. Available at http://www.aph.gov.au/hansard. The Standing Committee on Health and Ageing of the House of Representatives placed the Morris Enquiry report on record so that it was not lost from history.

Thomas H. Sick to death. Sydney: Allen and Unwin, 2007.

Final Report of the Queensland Public Hospitals Commission of Inquiry. (The Davies Report). Available at www.qphci.qld.gov.au. Accessed October 2010.

Medical Board of Queensland. Report to Gordon Nuttall MP on the registration of Dr Jayant Patel.

Australian Council for Safety and Quality in Healthcare. Standard for Credentialing and Defining Scope of Clinical Practice. Accessed July 2006 at http://www.safetyandquality.org/credentl.pdf

Walshe K, Shortell SM. When things go wrong: How healthcare organisations deal with major failures. Health Affairs 2004;23:103–111.

Queensland Health Systems Review. Final Report (the Forster Report). Accessed October 2010 at www.health.qld.gov.au

Prescription for trouble. About the House. Department of the House of Representatives. Issue 26, September 2006.

Barraclough BH, Birch, J. Healthcare safety and quality: where have we been and where are we going? Med JAust 2006;184,S48–S50.

Faunce TA, Bolsin, SNC. Three Australian whistleblowing sagas: lessons for internal and external regulation. Med JAust 2004;181,44–47.

Faunce T, Mure K, Cox C, Maher B. When silence threatens safety: lessons from the first Canberra Hospital neurosurgical inquiry. J Law Med 2004;12:112–118.

Morton, AP. Reflections on the Bundaberg Hospital failure. Med JAust 2005;183:328–329.

Van Der Weyden, MB. The Bundaberg Hospital scandal: the need for reform in Queensland and beyond (editorial), Med JAust 2005;183:284–285.

Barraclough, BH. Dramatic changes for the better are already occurring. Med JAust 2005;183:544.

Chapter 6

Gunderson JG, Ronningstam E. Differentiating narcissistic and antisocial personality disorders. J Personal Disord 2001;15:103–109.

Kernberg O. The narcissistic personality disorder and the differential diagnosis of antisocial behavior, Psychiatr Clin North Am 1989;12:553–570.

Hare RD, Without conscience: the disturbing world of psychopaths among us. New York: Pocket Books, 1993.

The Oregonian. PDF documents including results of Oregon medical Board reports, letters of praise from colleagues at Kaiser, job references, and letters of recommendation from Dr J Raymond Hinshaw of University of Rochester. Accessed 28 January 2007 at http://www.oregonlive.com/oregonian/malpractice/?/oregonian/malpractice/stories/storiesindex.html

Chapter 7

Thomas H. Sick to death. Sydney: Allen and Unwin, 2007.

The Oregonian. PDF documents including results of Oregon medical Board reports, letters of praise from colleagues at Kaiser, job references, and letters of recommendation from Dr J Raymond Hinshaw of University of Rochester. Unfortunately some of the links are now dead. Accessed 28 January 2007 at http://www.oregonlive.com/oregonian/malpractice/?/oregonian/malpractice/stories/storiesindex

Hansard. 16 March 2006. http://www.aph.gov.au/hansard. The Standing Committee on Health and Ageing of the House of Representatives placed the Morris Enquiry report on record so that it was not lost from history.

Final Report of the Queensland Public Hospitals Commission of Inquiry. (The Davies Report). Accessed October 2010 at www.qphci.qld.gov.au

Hare RD. *Without conscience: the disturbing world of psychopaths among us.* New York: Pocket Books, 1993

Clarke J. Working with monsters. Random House, 2005

Robert Kaplan on the *Health Report* 18 July 2005. Available at http://www.abc.net.au /rn/talks/8.30/helthrpt/stories/s1417427.htm

Sandall R. (Dec 2005, p. 12). Available at www.rogersandall.com/doctor-death-in-bund-aberg/

Chapter 8

Final Report of the Queensland Public Hospitals Commission of Inquiry. (The Davies Report). Available at www.qphci.qld.gov.au. Accessed October 2010

Bundaberg Hospital Commission of Inquiry. Transcript of Proceedings. Queensland Government Department of Justice and Attorney General, 23–26 May 2005 and www.casewatch.org

Hansard. 16 March 2006. http://www.aph.gov.au/hansard. The Standing Committee on Health and Ageing of the House of Representatives placed the Morris Enquiry report on record so that it was not lost from history.

Queensland Health Systems Review. Final Report (the Forster Report). Available at www.health.qld.gov.au. Accessed October 2010.

The Oregonian. PDF documents including results of Oregon medical Board reports, letters of praise from colleagues at Kaiser, job references, and letters of recommendation from Dr. J. Raymond Hinshaw of University of Rochester. Accessed 28 January 2007 at http://www.oregonlive.com/oregonian/malpractice/?/oregonian/malpractice/stories/storiesindex.html

Thomas H. Sick to death. Sydney: Allen and Unwin, 2007.

Chapter 9

Thomas H. Sick to death. Sydney: Allen and Unwin, 2007.

The Oregonian. PDF documents including results of Oregon Medical Board reports, letters of praise from colleagues at Kaiser, job references, and letters of recommendation from Dr J Raymond Hinshaw of University of Rochester. Unfortunately some of the links are now dead. Accessed 28 January 2007. http://www.oregonlive.com/oregonian/malpractice/?/oregonian/malpractice/stories/storiesindex

Hansard. 16 March 2006. http://www.aph.gov.au/hansard. The Standing Committee on Health and Ageing of the House of Representatives placed the Morris Enquiry report on record so that it was not lost from history.

Final Report of the Queensland Public Hospitals Commission of Inquiry. (The Davies Report). Accessed October 2010 at www.qphci.qld.gov.au

Queensland Health Systems Review. Final Report (the Forster Report). Accessed October 2010 at www.health.qld.gov.au

Australian Commission for Safety and Quality in Healthcare. Open disclosure. http://www.safetyandquality.gov.au/internet/safety/publishing.nsf/Content/Priority Program-02

Seven steps to patient safety. National Patient Safety Agency. Accessed October 2010 at http://www. nrls.npsa.nhs.uk/resources/collections/seven-steps-to-patient-safety/ and http://www.npsa.nhs.uk/site/media/documents/499_sevensteps_overview (2).pdf

Wimmera clinical risk management model — a systematic approach to reducing medical errors. Wimmera Healthcare Group, 2001.

Wolff AM, Bourke J, Campbell IA, Lambruggen D. Detecting and reducing hospital adverse events: outcomes of the Wimmera clinical risk management program MJA.

Craddick JW, Bader B. Medical management analysis: a systematic approach to quality assurance and risk management. Auburn, California: Joyce W. Craddick, 1983.

Nolan TW. System changes to improve patient safety. BMJ 2000;320:771–773.

Barraclough BH, Birch J. Healthcare safety and quality: where have we been and where are we going? Med J Aust 2006;184:S48–S50.

Wilson RM, Van Der Weyden M. The safety of Australian healthcare: 10 years after QAHCS. Med J Aust 2005;182:260–261.

Emslie S, Knox K, Pickstone M, eds. Improving patient safety: insights from American, Australian and British healthcare. London: ECRI &DH, 2002.

Vincent C. Incident reporting and patient safety. BMJ 2007; 334:51.

Van Der Weyden, MB, The Bundaberg Hospital scandal: the need for reform in Queensland and beyond (editorial). Med J. Aust 2005;183:284–285.

Walshe K, Shortell SM. When things go wrong: How healthcare organisations deal with major failures. Health Affairs 2004;23:103–111.

Livingston M, Woods, K. Evaluating clinical networks for cancer services in Scotland. Accessed October 2010 at http://www.integratedcarenetwork.org/publish/articles/000026/article_print.html

Mannion R, Davies HTO, Marshall MN. Cultures for performance in health care. New York: Open University Press, 2005.

Nelson EC, Batalden PB, Godfrey MM. Quality by design: a clinical microsystem approach. San Francisco: Jossey-Bass, 2007.

Rural Health Boards of Management Development Program. Workshop materials, produced for Department of Human Services Victoria by The Nous Group.

Chapter 10

Leape LL, Fromson JA. Problem doctors: is there a system-level solution? Ann Intern Med 2006;144:107–115.

Richard N, Pierson JR. In: Rosof AB, Felch WC, eds. Continuing medical education: A primer. Praeger 1992; 201–205.

Wilhelm KA, Reid AM. Critical decision points in the management of impaired doctors: the New South Wales Medical Board program. Med J Aust 2004;181:372–375.

Lehmann C. Mental illness sometimes overlooked in substance-abusing physicians. Psychiatric News 2004;39:11.

The Texas Medical Association Committee on Physician Health and Rehabilitation 2007. Accessed October 2010 at http://www.texmed.org

Diagnostic and Statistical Manual of Mental Disorders (DSM-IV-TR). American Psychiatric Association.

World Health Organization's International Classification of Diseases (ICD-10).

Hare RD. Without conscience: the disturbing world of psychopaths among us. New York: Pocket Books, 1993.

Gunderson JG, Ronningstam E. Differentiating narcissistic and antisocial personality disorders. J Personal Disord 2001;15:103–109.

Kernberg O. The narcissistic personality disorder and the differential diagnosis of anti-social behavior. Psychiatrc Clin North Am 1989;12:553–570.

Crow SM, Hartman SJ, Nolan TE, Zembo, M. A prescription for the rogue doctor. Part I – begin with diagnosis. Clinical Orthopaedics and Related Research 2003;411: 334–339.

Robert Kaplan on the Health Report 18 July 2005. Available at http://www.abc.net. au/rn/talks/8.30/helthrpt/stories/s1417427.htm

The Wall Street Journal about Swango's trial (19 July 2000).

Richard Neale: a career history. BBC news channel. Available at http://news.bbc.co.uk/ 1/hi/health/843594.stm

Professor accused of references. BBC news channel. Available at http://news.bbc. co.uk/1/hi/england/north_yorkshire/4484816.stm

Reeves G. ABC News. Accessed at http://search.abc.net.au/search/search.cgi?forM= simple&num_ranks=20&collection = abcall&query=graeme+reeves

Medical Errors Action Group. How MEAG export Graeme Reeves. Available at http://www.medicalerroraustralia.com/spotlight/butcher_of_bega.php

Walshe K, Shortell SM. When things go wrong: How healthcare organisations deal with major failures. Health Affairs 2004;23:103–111.

Seven steps to patient safety. National Patient Safety Agency. Accessed October 2010 at http://www.nrls.npsa.nhs.uk/resources/collections/seven-steps-to-patient-safety/; http://www.npsa.nhs.uk/site/media/documents/499_sevensteps_overview(2).pdf

Semmens JB, Aitken RJ, Sanfilippo FM, et al. The Western Australian Audit of Surgical Mortality: advancing surgical accountability. Med J Aust 2005;183:504-508.

Wolff A, Taylor S. Enhancing patient care: a practical guide to improving quality and safety in hospitals. Strawberry Hills, NSW: MJA Books, 2009.

Bent PD, Bolsin SN, Creati BJ, Colson ME. Professional monitoring and critical inci-dent reporting using personal digital assistants. Med J Aust 2002;177:496–499.

Barraclough BH, Birch J. Healthcare safety and quality: where have we been and where are we going? Med J Aust 2006;184:S48–S50.

Vincent C. Incident reporting and patient safety: emphasis is needed on measurement and safety improvement programs. BMJ 2007;334:51.

Chapter 11

Millenson M. Demanding medical excellence. Chicago: University of Chicago Press, 1997.

Principles for best practice in clinical audit. Accessed October 2010 at http://www.clingov.nscsha.nhs.uk/Default.aspx?aid=806

Halm EA, Lee C, Chassin MR. How is volume related to quality in healthcare? Annals of Internal Medicine 2002;137:511–520.

Coory MD, Baade PD. Urban-rural differences in prostate cancer mortality, radical prostatectomy and prostate specific antigen testing in Australia. Med J Austral 2005;182:112–115.

Hannan EL, Kilburn H, Racz M, Shields E, Chassin MR. Improving the outcomes of Coronary artery bypass surgery in New York State. JAMA 1994;271:761–766.

Berwick DM. A primer on leading improvement of systems. BMJ 1996;312:619–622.

Mannion R, Davies, HTO, Marshall, MN. Cultures for performance in health care. New York: Open University Press, 2005.

Nelson EC, Batalden PB, Godfrey MM. Quality by design: a clinical microsystem approach. San Francisco: Jossey-Bass, 2007.

Scally G, Donaldson LJ. Clinical governance and the drive for quality improvement in the new NHS in England. BMJ 1998;61–65.

Wolff AM, Taylor SA, McCabe JF. Using checklists and reminders in clinical pathways to improve hospital inpatient care. MJA 2004;181:428–431.

Wolff A, Taylor, S. Enhancing patient care: a practical guide to improving quality and safety in hospitals. Strawberry Hills, NSW: MJA Books, 2009.

Nolan, TW. System changes to improve patient safety. BMJ 2000;320:771–773.

Grol BMJ, Rubin GL, Frommer MS, Vincent NC, Phillips P, Leeder SR. Getting evidence into practice. Med JAust 2000;172:180–183.

Bent PD, Bolsin SN, Creati BJ, Colson ME. Professional monitoring and critical incident reporting using personal digital assistants. Med J Aust 2002;177:496–499.

Chapter 12

Final Report of the Queensland Public Hospitals Commission of Inquiry. (The Davies Report). Accessed October 2010 at www.qphci.qld.gov.au.

Queensland Health Systems Review. Final Report (the Forster Report). Accessed October 2010 at www.health.qld.gov.au

Loy CS, Warton RB, Dunbar JA. Workforce trends in specialist and GP obstetric practice in Victoria. Med J Austral 2007;186:26–30.

Maclean R, Bennet J. Nationally consistent assessment of international medical graduates. MJA 2008;188:464–468.

Australian Medical Council. Submission to the House of Representatives Joint Standing Committee on Migration. Accessed at http://www.aph.gov.au/house/committee/mig/recognition/subs/sub044.pdf

Mullan F. The metrics of the physician brain drain. NEJM 2005;353:1810–1818.

Arriving in Australia: overseas-trained doctors. Med JAust 2004;181:633–634.

Chapter 13

Courier-Mail, Brisbane. Accessed 13 October 2006 at http://blogs.news.com.au/courier-mail/vitalinterest/index.php/couriermail/comments/should_lavarch_have_brought_back_dr_patel/

The Australian. Accessed 16 October 2006 at http://www.theaustralian. com.au/news/nation/lavarch-misled-house-on-dr-death/story-e6frg6nf-1111112366185

Queensland Health. Six month health action plan checklist. Accessed at http://www. health.qld.gov.au/news/6mthchklist.asp

Duckett SJ. A new approach to clinical governance in Queensland. Australian Health Review; 2007:31.

Queensland Health Patient Safety Centre. Available at http://www. health.qld.gov. au/patientsafety/

Duckett SJ, Collins J, Maarten Kamp M, Walker K. An improvement focus in public reporting: The Queensland approach. Medical Journal of Australia 2008;189:616–617.

Queensland Health. Clinician performance support service. Available at http://www. health.qld.gov.au/clipss/

Good Medical Practice. General Medical Council, London. Accessed October 2010 at www.GMC-UK.org/guidance/good_medical_practice/index.ASP

Good Medical Practice. A code of conduct for doctors in Australia. Accessed at http://www.asa.org.au/static/_/2/243a676b2ef63f68572075ac5139d517.pdf

Van Der Weyden MB. Clinical senators. Medical Journal of Australia 2009;190:225.

Hansard. Accessed 16 March 2006 at http://www.aph.gov.au/hansard. The Standing Committee on Health and Ageing of the House of Representatives placed the Morris Inquiry report on record so that it was not lost from history.

Chapter 14

Barach P, Moss F. Delivering safe health care. BMJ 2001;323:585. doi: 10.1136/bmj. 323.7313.585

Kohn L, Corrigan J, Donaldson MS, eds. To err is human. Building a safer health system. Institute of Medicine. Washington DC: National Academy Press, 1999.

Wilson RM, RuncimanWB, Gibberd RW, Harrison BT, Newby L, Hamilton JD. The Quality in Australian Healthcare Study. Med J Aust 2001;163:458–71.

Leape LL. Human factors meets healthcare: the ultimate challenge. Ergonomics in design. 2004;12:6–12.

Dunbar JA, Reddy P. Beresford B, Ramsey WP, Lord RSA. In the wake of hospital inquiries: impact on staff and safety. Med J Aust 2007;186:80-83.

Douglas IN, Robinson J, Fahey K. Inquiry into Obstetric and Gynaecological Services at King Edward Memorial Hospital 1990-2000. Final Report: Government of Western Australia, 2001.

Special Commission of Inquiry into Campbelltown and Camden hospitals. Final Report: New South Wales Department of Health, 2004.

Child A, Glover P. Report on obstetric and gynaecological services at KEM and the Metropolitan Health Service Board, WA 2004.

Morton AP. Reflections on the Bundaberg Hospital failure. Med J Aust 2005;183: 328-329.

Van Der Weyden MB. The 'Cam affair': an isolated incident or destined to be repeated? (editorial). Med J Aust 2004;180:100–101.

Van Der Weyden MB. The Bundaberg Hospital scandal: the need for reform in Queensland and beyond (editorial). Med J Aust 2005;183:284–285.

Walshe K, Shortell SM. When things go wrong: How healthcare organisations deal with major failures. Health Affairs 2004;23:103–111.

An organisation with a memory: Department of Health, London. Accessed October 2010 at www.dh.gov.uk/publicationsandstatistics/publications/publicationspolicyandguidance.

Barraclough BH, Birch J. Healthcare safety and quality: where have we been and where are we going? Med J Aust 2006;184:S-48-S50.

Wilson RM, Van Dr Weyden M. The safety of Australian healthcare: 10 years after QAHCS. Med J Aust 2005;182:260-261.

Emslie S, Knox K, Pickstone M, eds. Improving patient safety: insights from American, Australian and British healthcare. London: ECRI &DH, 2002.

Reason J. Human error: models and management. BMJ 2000;320:768–770.

Westrum R. A typology of organisational cultures. Qual. Saf. Health Care 2004;13:22–27.

An organisation with a memory: Department of Health, London. Accessed October 2010 at www.dh.gov.uk/publicationsandstatistics/publications/publicationspolicyandguidance

Good Medical Practice. General Medical Council, London. Accessed October 2010 at www.GMC-UK.org/guidance/good_medical_practice/index.ASP

Referring a doctor to the GMC: a guide for individual doctors, medical directors and clinical governance managers. General Medical Council, London. Available at www.GMC-UK

Nolan TW. System changes to improve patient safety. BMJ 2000;320:771–773.

Seven steps to patient safety. National Patient Safety Agency. Accessed October 2010 at http://www.nrls.npsa.nhs.uk/resources/collections/seven-steps-to-patient-safety/ or http://www.npsa.nhs.uk/site/media/documents/499_sevensteps_overview(2).pdf

Scally G, Donaldson LJ. Clinical governance and the drive for quality improvement in the new NHS in England. BMJ 1998:61–65.

Smallwood RA. The safety and quality of healthcare: from Council to Commission. Med J Aust 2006;184:S39–S40.

Medical Board of Queensland. Report to Gordon Nuttall MP on the registration of Dr Jayant Patel.

Mannion R, Davies HTO, Marshall, MN. Cultures for performance in health care. New York: Open University Press, 2005.

Nelson EC, Batalden PB, Godfrey MM. Quality by design: a clinical microsystem approach. San Francisco: Jossey-Bass, 2007.

Duckett SJ. A new approach to clinical governance in Queensland. Australian Health Review, 2007;31:16–19.

Duckett SJ, Coory M, Sketcher-Baker, K. Identifying variation in the quality of care in Queensland hospitals. Med J Aust 2007;187:571–575.

Duckett SJ, Collins J, Kamp M, Walker K. An improvement focus on public health reporting: the Queensland approach. Med J Aust 2008;189:616–617.

The Report of the Public Inquiry into children's heart surgery at the Bristol Royal infirmary 1984-1995. Learning from Bristol. Accessed October 2010 at www.Bristol-inquiry.org.UK

BBC News, 2010, How the scandal developed. Accessed October 2010 at http://news.bbc.co.uk/2/hi/health/1218149.stm

Smith R. All changed, utterly changed. BMJ 1998;316:1917–1919.

Berwick DM. Not again! BMJ 2001;322:247–248.

Semmens JB, Aitken RJ, Sanfilippo FM, et al. The Western Australian Audit of Surgical Mortality: advancing surgical accountability. Med J Aust 2005;183:504–508.

Clinical Governance. Wikipedia. Accessed October 2010 at http://en.wikipedia.org/wiki/Clinical_Governance

Principles for Best Practice in Clinical Audit. Accessed at http://www.clingov.nscsha.nhs.uk/Default.aspx?aid=806

Ehsani JP, Jackson T, Duckett SJ. The incidence and cost of adverse events in Victorian hospitals 2003 to 2004. Med J Aust 2006;184: 551–555.

Vincent C. Incident reporting and patient safety: emphasis is needed on measurement and safety improvement programs. BMJ 2007;334:51.

Chapter 15

Graham C, 1994. Obituary Sir Roy Griffiths. The Independent. Accessed November 2010 at http://www.independent.co.uk/news/people/obituary-sir-roy-griffiths-1432347.html

Davies P. The Griffiths Report 25 years on. Health Service Journal 2009. Accessed November 2010 at http://www.hsj.co.uk/resource-centre/best-practice/the-griffiths-report-25-years-on/5001481.article

Thomas H. Sick to death. Sydney: Allen and Unwin, 2007.

Morris A, 2005. The black death in Queensland health. Speech to Queensland media club, 18 October 2005.

Morris A. Six myths about health care in Queensland, Queensland Master Builders Association.

Chapter 16

Magistrate rules Patel must remain in jail. Oregonian. 27 June 2008. Available at http://blog.oregonlive.com/breakingnews/2008/06/patel_hearing.html

Jayant Patel set for committal hearing. The Sunday Mail. Accessed 7 February 2009 at http://www.couriermail.com.au/news/queensland/patel-set-for-hearing/story-e6freoof-1111118786868

Decisions of the Nineteenth Century Tasmanian Superior Courts, published by the Division of Law, Macquarie University and the School of History and Classics,

University of Tasmania. Available at http://www.law.mq.edu.au/sctas/html/
1842cases/R%20v%20Valentine,%201842.htm

Seven years jail for Jayant Patel. News Mail, 1 July 2010. Available at http://www.news-
mail.com.au/story/2010/07/01/jayant-patel-sentenced-manslaughter/

Chapter 17

The triumph of hope over experience. NHS Confederation. Available at www.nhscon-
fed.org

Oxman AD, Sackett DL, Chalmers I, Prescott TE. A surrealistic mega analysis of redisor-
ganisation theories. J R Soc Med 2005;98:563–568.

Coid D, Davies H. Healthcare workers well being and therapeutic relationship: does
organisational change to damage? Public Money and Management, 2007.

Coid D, Davies H. Structural change in healthcare: what's the attraction? J R Soc Med
2008;101:278–281.

Braithwaite G, Westbrook J, Iedema R. J R Soc Med 2005;98:542–544

Beattie must not shift the blame to others. The Australian. 27 July 2010.

Http://www.theaustralian.com.au/news/opinion/beattie-must-not-shift-blame-to-
others/story-e6frg6zo-1225888686946

Health Consumers Queensland. http://www.health.qld.gov.au/hcq/default.asp

Queensland Health Patient Safety Centre. http://www.health.qld.gov.au/patientsafety/

Index